CAMELIA PANATI

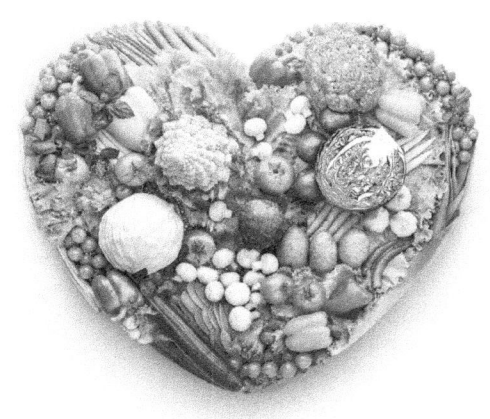

YOUR HEALTHY ZESTY *Life*

6 STEPS FOR OVERCOMING EXHAUSTION AND ACHIEVING VIBRANT HEALTH!

Your Healthy Zesty Life

6 Steps for Overcoming Exhaustion and Achieving Vibrant Health!

Copyright © 2016 by CAMELIA PANATI

Images used under license Shutterstock.com

To contact the author, visit
www.healthyzesty.com

ISBN-13: 978-1539516781

Printed in the United States of America

First and foremost, I dedicate this book to my loving and cherished daughter, Alexa, who has been my biggest supporter and cheerleader throughout the years and my biggest reason to keep up the fight and heal myself. She has always believed in me and my ability to help and inspire others live a healthy and vibrant life! She is the center of my universe and my best, unconditional, friend! I hope she will carry on my legacy by continuing to follow the sound principles for a healthy and vibrant life highlighted in this book.

Last, but not least, this book wouldn't have been a reality without the unconditional support of my loving husband, Razvan, who has been next to me and cared for me every step of the way during and past my health crisis. He has been a witness to my suffering, but also to my miraculous recovery, which is why he continues to encourage me to follow my passion of spreading the word about the importance of healthy eating and balanced living for a healthy and happy life!

But above all, this book was written with a heart full of love and gratitude and the intention to inspire you, my dear reader, to live a healthy, happy and vibrant life!

Table of Contents

Part One

My Story

MY STORY

Introduction

I believe we should all feel vibrant and healthy in order to live a happy life and become the best version of ourselves! Too often we find ourselves giving up on our dreams, on our life goals because we don't have the stamina, energy or motivation to keep on going and reaching for what makes us truly happy and complete.

Have you ever wondered why others reach those heights in life that seem unattainable to us, and why they always seem to be in a good mood and ready to take over the world? "What are they having?" you wonder, "I'll have that, too", you'd say; only if that were something you could order with a snap.

I'll let you in on a little secret here. You can have that attitude and better chances to reaching your goals. The 6 steps outlined in this book will help you change the way you think, the way you eat and the way you care for yourself. Those people who seem to have it all together, although maybe unconsciously, are doing most of these things right without even realizing it. It may be second nature, education or acquired skills, or a combination. They have the right attitude, they know that their own persona is a priority, they eat healthily and exercise, they know building and maintaining healthy relationships is as important, and they do work that they love. And on top of it all, they have a purpose!

Sounds trivial, right? Well, it's not that common sense to most of us. I know it wasn't for me before I hit rock bottom and it took me a while to put everything together and realize the importance of all these things that make us whole and shape who we are and how we feel.

MY STORY

The Wake-up Call

Any change begins as a result of a life experience, whether that's positive or negative. There needs to be a powerful driving force or motive for that change to actually grow roots and become part of our life, part of who we are today. It's part of human evolution.

And boy, did I evolve.

Four years ago, I was working as a Director of Risk in the payments industry when my health took a major turn. I struggled with not having the energy to perform the simplistic of tasks. But the most devastating toll was the quality time I lost with my little one. To play with her without feeling exhausted, or experiencing throbbing headache, became a chore.

On top of my exhaustion, my digestion was always in disarray. Eating a meal was like playing Russian Roulette with my stomach. Would I get indigestion? Gas pains? Feel more sluggish than I already was? Like I needed that. I chalked it up to what everyone with a career and family goes through: aging.

But my symptoms got worse. I woke up in the middle of the night more anxious about my health, worrying about who was going to take care of my little one if something terrible were to happen to me.

So, I followed my instinct and went to see my gastroenterologist doctor again: "I know there is something wrong with me. I don't know what it is, but I am not feeling like myself", I said.

That visit to the doctor, that instinct to listen to my gut feeling, saved my life! It turned out I had colon cancer at the early age of 38. And that's how my journey to a healthy-zesty life started. That was the event, the life experience that changed my life and led me on the path to a Healthy-Zesty life! Now, I want to help you take control over your health and life. With the knowledge I've learned from my own experience, I can teach you how to make gradual nutritional and lifestyle shifts that will infuse you with energy and zest for life!

Once that happens, don't be surprised to hear people around you saying "I'll have what she's having!"

Path to Redemption

I won't lie to you. The journey was not easy at first. For years I struggled with digestive distress, headaches, brain fog and lack of energy. I felt I was actually missing out on life, missing out on experiencing the beauty and wonders life has to offer when you live in the present and are in-tune with your higher self. But I was too busy to complain and just went with the flow, hoping that tomorrow things would get better. If or when I got that promotion, if or when I got more money, when my daughter would grow up... things would get better and I'd focus on my health. I felt I was too young to let all these symptoms get in my way. I was even ashamed to admit that I was feeling older on the inside than my driver's license dared to reveal. So, I kept looking for quick fixes that would allow me to get a bit of a boost in energy, convincing myself that what I was feeling was just temporary exhaustion. And maybe it was... until things got worse.

I had to hit rock bottom in order to realize this was no temporary exhaustion. Not anymore. The cancer was eating me on the inside and I couldn't let that happen.

My priorities shifted overnight. In order to achieve what I wanted professionally and as a mother I had to first heal myself, find that balance I was lacking and finally get my life back. I had to learn to make myself a priority, to listen to my body, nurture my body and soul and finally live a healthy-zesty life!

And while it took me a few years of trial and error to come to this realization and simplify my recovery into the steps outlined in this book, it is my hope that my story will be a wake-up call for you, too. By following my "6 steps for overcoming exhaustion and achieving vibrant health" for looking and feeling your best, you too will be able to finally live a healthy-zesty life! It's really not that hard. You just need to identify the why behind feeling healthy and vibrant. Because feeling healthy and vibrant is just the enabler, the tool that will get you where you want in life. It's not the final destination.

So, back to you now: What is that you really want? Why do you want to feel healthy and vibrant? What's in this for you? What's your deep down motivation?

The answers to these questions are going to keep you motivated on your path to living a healthy-zesty life!

 Make note of these questions and answers and revisit them whenever you are falling off track. Don't be surprised if the answers will change over time. It's not unusual for that to happen as you advance in the program and get more clarity over your goals in life.

A Blessing in Disguise?

On my path to healing, I started looking for answers from my doctors first. While they did a great job identifying and removing the evil that was inside me, they failed to answer my "why, how and what now?" Because, although I was cancer free, I was still feeling sick.

I decided that it was time for me to fight for my own health and do all I could to prevent the cancer from coming back. I started my own journey of researching possible root causes and holistic cures for colon cancer and digestive issues and ended up changing my diet and my life for the better.

Only a couple of weeks after I changed my diet I felt like a veil came off my eyes and I suddenly felt awake, focused and energized. I knew this is what a healthy body should feel like. Within a year I had progressively restored my digestive balance, improved my alertness and felt alive again.

My desire to be around for my little one is what motivated me to keep looking and become my own educator for living a healthy, vibrant and purposeful life. That's what led me to deepen my own research for holistic healing and enrolled into the Institute for Integrative Nutrition® (IIN®) in New York, the largest Nutrition school in the world. Thanks to IIN, I learned not only how to properly feed my body for health and energy, but also how to practice self-care, both very important in achieving that special balance between body, mind, and soul and therefore, overall wellbeing.

My own journey, my new found passion for holistic health and balanced living, was what led me to make a major career change, too. I realized I stumbled upon something big. Something that had the potential of helping many others overcome their own chronic health problems and finally enjoy vibrant health. That's why I call this event that changed my life, a blessing in disguise.

I took a break from my corporate job, which was for me poisoning at the time, and launched my own Holistic Health Coaching Practice. That's how "**Healthy Zesty Path to Wellness**" was born!

I now feel healthy, happy and alive, and I want to share this state of wellbeing with others.

My purpose is to share this knowledge and practice with the world and help you, my dear reader, live a healthy and vibrant life that will enable you to do what you love!

We only have one life to live, so we better make the best of it!

Visit www.healthyzesty.com for even more information!

MY STORY

Path to Healthy Zesty Living

What is a healthy-zesty life?

Healthy = the physical and spiritual state that makes us feel whole and allows us to go after our dreams

Zesty = vibrant, passionate, desirable and ready to enjoy life to its fullest

In my opinion, living a healthy-zesty life means living the life you were meant to live. Living a life that allows you to become the best version of yourself while feeling healthy and vibrant and ready to conquer the world. Being ready for the next big step without being held back by feelings of exhaustion, sluggishness, lack of clarity or motivation. Because no matter how much you want to achieve that special something in life, chances are you will struggle to find your way through if your energy levels are down or you are bothered by other chronic health issues.

For me personally, healthy-zesty life means being cancer free, feeling full of energy to spend quality time with my family, do work I love and travel the world, all while looking vibrant and living life with purpose!

I am going to let you in on a little secret here: up until 3 years ago, I didn't know what my purpose was. Even after I recovered from my own health problems, when I thought I was ok, I was still not completely ok. I knew I was missing something. I knew there had to be more to life than what I was living. But I just didn't know what. I didn't have the clarity and self-awareness needed to find my purpose. To find that joy that would make life more exciting. Of course, I was happy I was alive and cancer free. But now, after the experience I had been through, I knew I had to make my life worth living. I knew that what happened was for a reason. So I started to listen to my internal signals and asked myself often, "What is my higher purpose?"

I am telling you this because finding your purpose, doing what you love and living a healthy-zesty life, starts with self-awareness. And self-awareness is not something you develop overnight. It's something you cultivate over time with practice. Becoming more self-aware will be one of the side effects experienced once you start implementing the steps outlined later on in the book, in part 3.

You won't know if you are living the life of your dreams unless you know what that looks like to you. So, defining that is the first step in measuring your present state and developing an action plan for achieving your future goal.

But this is not all. Getting where you need or want to be and feeling your best requires that you have the energy it takes to reach your goal and truly enjoy it. What's the point in getting to travel the most exotic parts of the world if your health is poor and your energy is down?

You see, you can't have one without the other. Which is why feeling healthy and vibrant is just the enabler, not the destination. This, my friend, should be your number one priority on the path to a healthy-zesty life!

Why the Healthy-Zesty Diet is not a Diet, but a Lifestyle

You're probably wondering, what is a healthy-zesty diet? Well, it's not truly a diet, but more so a lifestyle. It's not something that you need to keep up with for a few weeks and then go back to your old eating habits. That is yo-yo dieting and I'm sure you had enough of that so far, which is why you got this book in the first place. My goal is to help you make gradual shifts in your eating habits, such that the changes made will stick for the rest of your life. My goal is for you to be one of the adopters of the healthy-zesty lifestyle, which is what this book is all about. Just don't think of it as a diet, because it is not. And you will understand later on why that is.

Because of the limitations of fad diets and drawing on the knowledge acquired during my search for answers and during my holistic nutrition studies, I developed my own healthy diet based on trial and error practices I experienced myself. This is what I like to call the healthy-zesty diet. What's different, though, is that this is not a diet, but a life-style. The healthy-zesty diet discussed throughout the book should be seen as a guide for building new healthy habits to last a lifetime.

My hope is that this book will be an eye-opener for you, and it will help you understand the main message I want to convey: **that a healthy-zesty diet is not truly a diet, it is a way of living your life in order to enjoy vibrant health and look and feel your best!**

My Approach

Just like I tell my clients in my holistic health coaching practice (see **Healthy Zesty Path to Wellness** at www.healthyzesty.com), my approach is not focused on following a strict diet, but more so on bio-individuality. One person's food could be another person's poison![1] Which is why I focus on helping clients identify what works for them, what motivates them, what gives them the energy and zest for life and can be easily integrated into their lifestyle, such that the changes made last for a lifetime.

I am a big believer in the **healing power of whole foods**. Like one of my teachers, Joshua Rosenthal, used to say, "*You give your body what it needs to heal itself, by itself.*" If we tune in and learn to listen to our body, we intuitively know to give it what is best. It takes time, practice and support. And that's where my help comes in handy. I will guide you, provide useful and actionable advice that will support you in

---

1 © 2007 Integrative Nutrition Inc. (used with permission)

making gradual and sustainable lifestyle changes in line with your ultimate goal of being and feeling like the best version of yourself!

As I said, I don't believe one diet fits all, which is why we should all be flexible in our approach to food to some degree. Otherwise, we could quickly fall off track and switch from extremely healthy eating to binge eating and uncontrollable cravings. I am, therefore, a big supporter of *Joshua's 90-10 Diet*,[2] meaning eat right most of the time and allow yourself the liberty of being somewhat "bad" at times. As a result of my approach, not only will you not feel you are on a diet, but your cravings – which is what usually sabotages our healthy eating efforts – will gradually disappear.

More importantly, as you will see in part 3 where I offer actionable advice, I put a lot of emphasis on **digestive health**, as I am a living proof of the devastating effects an unbalanced gut could have on your overall health. You probably heard before that "happiness comes from within" and believe me, that is literally your Gut! **The Gut is responsible for your overall wellbeing!** Your Gut sits at the core of your mental and physical health and has a huge impact on your health and vitality.

Last, but not least, it's vitally important not only what you feed your physical body, but also how you nurture your whole self. Which brings my focus on another important aspect of overall healing and well-being: Self Care. You will be mesmerized by the impact the combination of proper nutrition and self-care has on your overall wellbeing and outlook on life.

---

2 ©2008 Integrative Nutrition Inc. (used with permission)

My hope is that by following the advice in this book you will be able to discover what is missing from your life and how you can bring back balance – a necessary practice for overall wellbeing.

As you can see, the main pillars of a healthy-zesty diet focus not only on nutrition but lifestyle and self-care as well. This type of approach will make you understand the importance of **healthy eating and balanced living**, which is what we all need in order to live a healthy and zesty life.

Based on this integrative approach, I want to make you understand that although we are made from what we eat, **our whole self and wellbeing is the result of a multitude of factors, such as experiences, career, relationships, spirituality, community, physical exercise and of course nutrition.** All these shape who we are and how we feel. Therefore, with the help of this book and by following the 6 actionable steps outlined in part 3 you will be prompted to reflect on every aspect of your life that could potentially affect how you eat and ultimately feel. The transformations I've seen so far in my practice as a result of my one on one coaching interactions based on the same pillars have been amazing! Take this book as a mini private coaching program, without the personal interaction and accountability and without the expense. However, if you feel you need that special personal attention, accountability and a program tailored specifically to your own needs, you can always reach out to me at cameliapanati@healthyzesty.com or you can check out my website: www.healthyzesty.com.

Part Two

The 6 Steps to a Healthy Zesty Life

THE STEPS

Introduction

During my studies at the Institute for Integrative Nutrition®, I was first introduced to the concept of the Circle of Life [3] which encompasses all aspects that could affect one's well-being: food, self-care, relationships, career, physical exercise and spirituality. It is the balance between all these things that will help us achieve ideal health, weight, and overall wellbeing. And when you are healthy, balanced and full of energy you are happy and ready to go live life with purpose.

So you see, that's why I say that feeling healthy and vibrant is not the final goal, but the enabler, what will take you to your actual goal and destination. If you are not healthy and you feel sluggish and unhappy chances are you won't be able to get that promotion, or find the love of your life, or travel the world, or find your purpose, or achieve whatever dream you have.

The purpose of this book is to bring awareness around what is that impacts the way you feel and look and your overall wellbeing; awareness around the secret formula to living a healthy-zesty life, according to my definition.

3 © Integrative Nutrition Inc. (Used with permission)

The principles of a healthy-zesty life are based on six fundamental pillars that when interrelated make us whole and bring us into balance. And when we are balanced we feel and look vibrant!

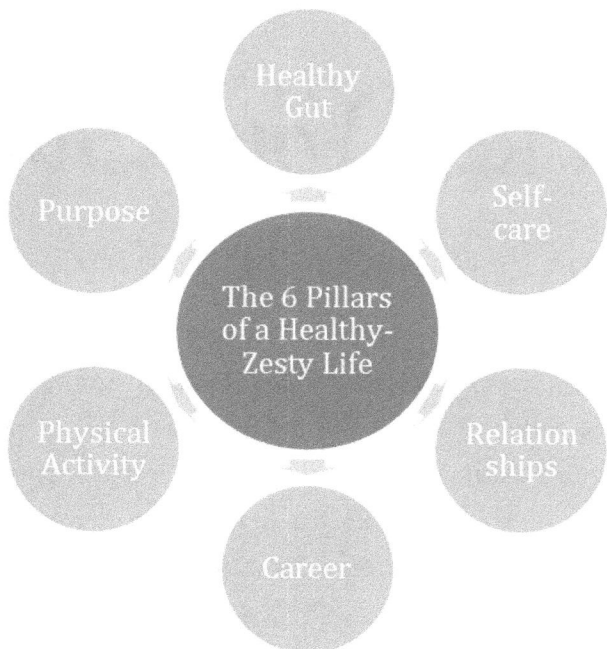

These six pillars sit at the foundation of the 6 steps program I developed for overcoming exhaustion and achieving vibrant health. I invite you to read through, take notes and start implementing the recommendations as you progress through the book. However, as you finish reading the book, I encourage you to take a moment to draw your own conclusions, reflect over where you are in the healing process, what you still need to improve upon and identify your next steps needed for implementing what you learned for living a healthy-zesty life.

The 6 steps outlined throughout the book will help you achieve balance, improve your energy, lose weight, boost your mood and overall wellbeing and get you ready for becoming the best version of yourself and living the life you were meant to live. Get ready for uncovering a healthy, zesty you! Get ready for your own transformation!

STEP ONE

Heal Your Gut

Happiness comes from within. No, really. It literally comes from your Gut! **The Gut is responsible for your overall wellbeing.** Your gut sits at the core of your mental and physical health and has a huge impact on your health and vitality. It directly impacts your mood, energy, and weight. That's why it's the first and most important step in regaining your energy and living a healthy and zesty life.

When your Gut is out of balance, not only is your digestion compromised, but it triggers inflammation in your body, which in turn brings upon a multitude of inflammation-related health problems. These include, but are not limited to, Irritable Bowel Syndrome (IBS) or other digestive ailments, depression, weight gain, migraines, autoimmune diseases, fatigue, fogginess, food allergies and sensitivities, all the way to cancers.

According to a survey published by Fox News in 2013, about 74% of Americans suffer from digestive discomfort. [4] While these people know that their discomfort is tummy related, there are way more undiagnosed patients suffering from Gut imbalance related illnesses without

4 (FoxNews.com)

even knowing it. Just because you don't have a tummy ache it doesn't mean your Gut is in perfect health. The conditions mentioned above are all related to some kind of Gut imbalance. You will see that by restoring your Gut health, other inflammatory conditions in your body will improve as well.

The health of our Gut is influenced by both internal and external factors. The internal factors are really based on what we put into our bodies, our diet, while the external factors could be stress, relationships, environment, pesticides and chemicals we breathe in or even ingest as part of our diet without even knowing. I call these Hidden Evils.

But the biggest evil of all is our SAD diet. The Standard American Diet full of refined carbs and sugars. That's what makes us sad, indeed!

According to Mayo Clinic's Center for Innovation, only about 12% of Americans manage to eat the recommended servings of fruits and vegetables based on the government recommended diet – which, in my opinion, is still a far fetch from a truly healthy diet – while the majority of us eat the SAD diet.[5]

The study reveals that more than half of a typical American's diet is made up of processed foods, such as refined carbs, sugars, artificial sweeteners and packaged foods. This is what strips away your Gut flora making room for inflammation that could trigger a series of other ailments in your body.

_____

5 (Keefe)

The Gut – Brain Connection

There is a strong body of evidence regarding the connection between the Gut and the brain. Research shows that the composition of our microbiome – the collection of microbes and bacteria found in our Gut – could impact how we feel. That would explain why when we eat a diet full of sugars and refined carbs we are left feeling spacey, tired and later on depressed.

Aside from mood, the Gut also impacts our level of focus, clarity, and alertness. There is no surprise the Gut is now considered our second brain. Researchers suggest that there are more neurons in our Gut than there are in the spinal cord or the peripheral nervous system (over 100 million neurons).

Those butterflies of emotion we feel when we fall in love are a result of these nerves in our Gut. Stress, too, is processed through the Gut, as a result of the gut-brain connection. This explains why we get ulcers, gastritis or just plain old stomach aches when we are nervous and overly stressed. Even more, some researchers argue that certain depression treatments that target the mind could inadvertently impact our gut health. [6] You will soon understand that, due to this gut-brain connection, by reducing stress you will improve digestion and by improving digestion you will improve your mental health.

6 (Hadhazy)

The Good and the Bad in Your Gut

About 70% of our immune system is located in the Gut. As a result, more microbes and bacteria are found in the Gut than in the rest of the body. What we eat directly impacts the composition of the microbiome and thus our immune system. It is important that we maintain a healthy balance of the good (beneficial) bacteria versus bad bacteria, in order for our Gut to function properly (about 85 to 15 ratio is ideal, although the more good bacteria the better).

The good bacteria is friendly to us and helps our gut stay happy and healthy, whereas the bad bacteria is not friendly at all, it actually eats away our intestinal friends. So the more friends you make on the inside, the better chances you have to win the war against the intestinal enemies! And the goal is not only to make friends but to nourish and maintain them as well; just like you do with relationships in real life.

To make more intestinal friends you need to eat more probiotic promoting foods and less of the gut hurting foods, such as refined carbs and sugars. To maintain the great friends you made you need to treat them well, so they grow bigger and don't run away. You need to nourish them with dietary fiber from plants and prebiotics like inulin, psyllium, and other non-digestible dietary fiber that not only feeds the friendly bacteria but helps you properly digest food and move it smoothly down the colon and into the toilet.

Top 6 Disruptors of the Gut Balance

Even if we are nice to our intestinal friends and let them in through supplements and enriched foods, we still need to protect them from getting washed-out by the bad guys. Our Gut gets depleted of beneficial bacteria as a result of:

❈ Chronic stress

❈ Recurring use of antibiotics and steroids (even one round of antibiotic a year wreaks havoc on our digestive system)

❈ Chemicals and pesticides found in our food or environment

❈ Excessive consumption of refined sugars and carbs (white flour, white sugar, high fructose corn syrup)

❈ Excessive alcohol consumption

❈ Artificial sweeteners

Steps for Improving Your Gut Health

In the next several pages I am going to walk you through a series of action steps meant to improve your Gut health and boost your energy and alertness as a result. As I mentioned before, healing your gut is the first and maybe most important step on the path to overcoming exhaustion and achieving vibrant health. Therefore, implementing these action steps for healing your gut will have the biggest impact on your overall wellbeing. I suggest you start implementing each of these action steps as soon as you've made yourself familiar with the content and had a chance to plan your shopping list accordingly. By taking one step at a time as you progress through the book, your transition will be smoother and will help you feel supported along the way. Although I am not there with you in person, please know that I wrote this book with you, my dear reader, in mind. I wrote this book to coach you, support you and hold you accountable on your path to becoming the best version of yourself and living the life you were meant to live.

You know already that you were meant for better things. You know that your life should not be reduced to feeling sick and tired all the time, with no zest for life. I am here to reassure you that you are right. You have the right to feel healthy and vibrant and should not settle for anything less than that. So, brace yourself and get ready for a happy gut and a healthy-zesty you!

The foundation of my approach to improving gut health is the 4R Program developed by Dr. Jeffrey Bland, Ph.D.: remove, replace, re-inoculate and repair. [7]

---

7 (Lipman)

Drawing on this approach, I put together the following sequence of action steps for restoring gut health and preparing your body to function at its best:

1. CLEAN OUT YOUR PLATE

- Remove food iritants
- Eliminate toxic load

2. EAT WHOLE

- Crowd-out bad stuff
- Add in good stuff

3. HYDRATE

- Drink plenty of water

4. REBALANCE INTESTINAL FLORA

- Promote beneficial bacteria (probiotics)
- Nourish beneficial bacteria (prebiotics)

5. SUPPORT DIGESTION

- Take digestive enzymes
- Eat natural bitters

6. GET COOKING

- Experiment with home cooked meals

7. SUPPLEMENT WITH GUT HEALING NATURAL SUPPLEMENTS

- Quercetine
- L-gluthamine

8. REPLAY

- Repeat the process anually

HEAL YOUR GUT - ACTION STEP 1

Clean Out Your Plate

Cleaning out your plate consists of removing food irritants and reducing toxic load.

Remove Food Irritants

This is the most important stage in restoring your Gut health, as removing foods known to create digestive distress and impact the way you feel day in - day out will give you a fresh start in rebalancing your Gut and gaining that state of wellbeing you have been craving for.

Remember: **your gut sits at the core of your mental and physical health; what you eat directly impacts how you feel and look.** Once your gut is optimally balanced, your energy, too, will be improved.

Foods to be removed from your diet completely for at least 2 weeks:

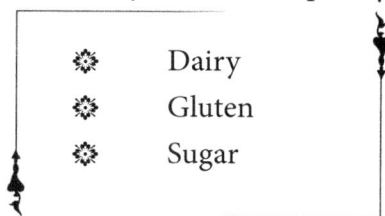

❋ Dairy

❋ Gluten

❋ Sugar

These food groups are known to create inflammation in the body, thus making us feel tired, bloated and foggy when eaten in excess.

This might sound a bit intimidating but please don't despair, you will be able to enjoy these food groups again. Although, preferably in a more unrefined and whole form. Trust me, although you must feel a bit discouraged now, your body and especially your gut will feel relieved to be getting a break from the aggravating effects these foods have on them.

Before starting the 2 weeks elimination I recommend you read through the next few pages to identify what it is that you need to avoid and what you have to stock up your pantry and fridge with, so you don't give in to temptation due to lack of better choices. You need to find healthier alternatives to foods you used to eat before to make the transition smoother and to fool your brain while satisfying your craving. This is the key to sticking with a healthy diet.

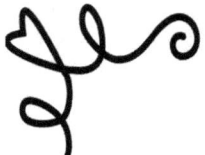

Benefits of Removing Food Irritants

As hard as it may seem to give up on these food groups at first, hang in there! There are lots of goodies happening in your body during this time and you will be able to enjoy most of these benefits at the end of the elimination stage:

- Immediate boost in energy
- Improved digestion
- Clear thinking
- Better mood
- Fewer headaches
- Sinus decongestion
- Clear skin
- Weight loss
- Improved alertness
- Better control over cravings
- Uncovering food triggers and sabotaging habits
- Reduced allergy symptoms
- Reduced occurrence of food sensitivities

Withdrawal Symptoms

You know the saying – "no pain, no gain". Well, as much as you might dislike it, this holds true for this stage of the program, too. Just like with any detox, when your body is highly used to a certain habit or food, refraining from it may trigger some withdrawal symptoms. It is more common to experience some withdrawal symptoms, when removing gluten and sugar. That's because both gluten and sugar are addicting and habit forming, a stronger reason for you to detox your body and get back control over your cravings.

It's a vicious cycle, the more you crave a certain food group (such as sugar, gluten or even dairy) the more your body is addicted to it. Some people do experience mild withdrawal symptoms a couple of days after being completely gluten and sugar-free and they typically subside within a few days. This varies from person to person and depends on the extent to which you depended on those foods.

These foods also increase the chances of you having a slight sensitivity. So pay attention to what is the most difficult for you to give up to during these 2 weeks of abstinence and be mindful of how your body reacts when you reintroduce that food into your diet for the first time after the elimination period. I suggest keeping a food journal as you remove and reintroduce these foods back into your diet. Doing so will give you valuable insight into potential food sensitivity, which I discuss later on in the Reintroduction Stage.

Here are some of the withdrawal symptoms that could be experienced on a detox, so don't you freak out if you end up experiencing any of them – just know that things will look up and the benefits outweigh the temporary drawbacks:

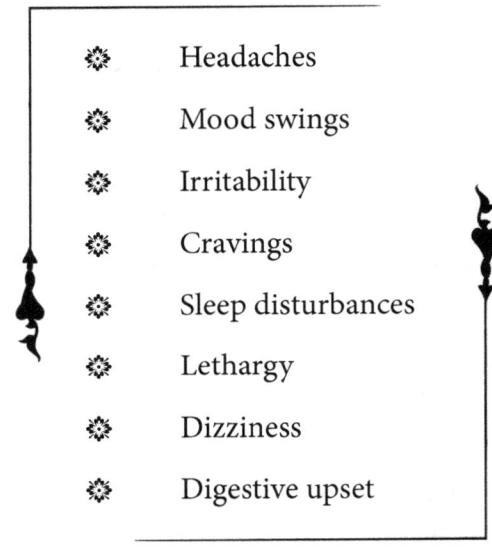

❁ Headaches

❁ Mood swings

❁ Irritability

❁ Cravings

❁ Sleep disturbances

❁ Lethargy

❁ Dizziness

❁ Digestive upset

Rest assured that you won't experience all of these symptoms. You might very well not deal with any of these symptoms at all!

Tips For Easing in the Elimination Stage

Use transition foods

Some examples are gluten-free bread, gluten-free flours, agave syrup, dairy-free cheese, and tofu. For instance, if you are used to eating bread, stock up on gluten-free bread before you start the elimination period. Same goes for sugar – if you are used to adding sugar to your morning coffee, have the sugar substitutes, such as agave syrup, handy. If dairy is a big thing for you, use substitutes such as rice milk, coconut milk, dairy-free cheese (read the labels for other harmful ingredients, such as carrageenan, and even gluten).

Clean-up your pantry

By removing the "offenders" from your pantry you will be less likely to fall into temptation and cravings. And you know who those offenders are – sugar, wheat products, packaged foods and any overly processed foods that are laden with sugars, gluten, and trans fats. I suggest you clean up your pantry before you start the elimination and make room for some healthy snacks.

Stock up on healthy snacks

In order to curb cravings you need to not be starving! Have some healthy snacks handy at all times. Pack snacks for work, add some in your handbag to have them handy in case your blood sugar drops. Healthy snacks suggestions: mini carrots, celery sticks with hummus, nuts (go nuts about nuts – they are good for you as they are a good source of protein and rich in healthy fats), fresh fruits (especially berries), roasted seaweed, nut butter with apple slices or gluten-free crackers.

Practice deep breathing exercises

Deep breathing helps you center yourself, relaxes your mind and body and supports digestion. By implementing this into your daily routine you will cope better with the angst you might feel at first when going off sugar and gluten. My favorite breathing practice is the 4-7-8 exercise I learned from Dr. Andrew Weil, M.D., one of the visiting teachers at the Institute for Integrative Nutrition®, whom I respect dearly. Dr. Weil is a big promoter of the anti-inflammatory diet and is known as a guru in the holistic and integrative medicine. [8]

How to practice the 4-7-8 breathing exercise

Place the tip of your tongue on the gum ridge of your upper teeth and inhale deeply while counting to 4; hold it for 7 counts and release it during 8 counts. Repeat this up to 4 times. You might have a lightheaded feeling at the end, especially in the beginning if breathing exercises are a new practice to you.

By doing this practice regularly not only will you calm down your mind and digestive system, but you will ease your cravings and get an overall sense of wellbeing.

Tongue scrub

This is an Ayurveda tradition for mouth health. It removes deposits built up on the tongue, which eliminates bad breath and the development of bacteria in the mouth. But what I find even more interesting is that the tongue scrub helps fight food cravings, as the food we used to eat doesn't remain on the taste buds and thus we don't feel like we have to eat it over and over again. Additionally, by keeping a clean tongue we get to better taste the different flavors in our food, making us more

8 (DrWeil.com)

likely to enjoy the taste of healthier options.

You can find a tongue scraper online or in special health stores. I got mine on Amazon and I use it regularly, morning and evening after brushing my teeth.

Gluten

Gluten is the protein found in grains, such as wheat, barley, and rye. It is what gives baked foods the doughy structure.

While people suffering from celiac disease or a wheat allergy must avoid gluten at all costs, people reporting sensitivity to gluten might benefit from ditching the gluten as well. Though their life is not endangered by the consumption of occasional gluten.

Gluten sensitivity occurs when your body has a harder time digesting the protein found in gluten, called gliadin. The immune system negatively reacts to it by attacking the gluten protein just like it would a foreign invader and thus an inflammatory process takes place. As a result, the following symptoms could occur:

❈ Upper and lower GI issues: indigestion, bloating, heartburn, excessive burping, diarrhea, excessive gas, constipation
❈ Foggy mind
❈ Headaches
❈ Reduced alertness and energy
❈ Joint pains.

Therefore, you should avoid consuming any foods containing gluten for at least 2 weeks in order to give your digestive system a break from the inflammatory effects it could have on your body.

Foods to Avoid [9]

- Wheat
- Kamut
- Spelt
- Rye
- Barley
- Oats are generally avoided because they are almost always processed in mills that process grains containing gluten. Look for gluten-free oats.
- Modified food starch
- Barley enzymes (found in majority of breakfast cereals), soy sauce, and distilled vinegar (malt vinegar)
- Soy sauce typically contains gluten (look for tamarind sauce, which is the gluten-free version of traditional soy sauce)

9 © Integrative Nutrition Inc.(used with permission)

Gluten-Free Foods [10]

❋ Potatoes

❋ Buckwheat

❋ Oats (*must be labeled gluten-free to avoid cross-contamination)

❋ Corn/ maize

❋ Rice

❋ Quinoa

❋ Amaranth

❋ Teff

❋ Millet

❋ Beans

❋ Nuts and nuts butter

❋ Eggs

❋ Fresh fruit

❋ Fresh vegetables

❋ Herbs and spices

❋ Meats and fish purchased without sauce or seasonings

❋ Home-made soups (avoid bouillon cubes, barley malt, and all types of pasta, unless they are labeled gluten-free)

❋ Juice (all-natural, 100% fruit juice)

10 © Integrative Nutrition Inc.(used with permission)

Dairy

Dairy is another food group that is known to have an inflammatory effect on your body when consumed in excess. Just like gluten, dairy too can cause allergies, but more often than not, people could develop a sensitivity to it without even knowing. And that's probably because, just like gluten and sugar, dairy is found in almost every packaged or baked food.

Since we consume it so often, our body gets tired of it and has a harder time digesting it properly and starts fighting back. Think of how you react personally to a food you are sick and tired of and don't feel like eating it anymore (whether that's the green beans your mom kept telling you to eat as a child or something else you had too much of). You try to push that food aside and don't even bother to chew. So does your digestive system when it comes to digesting something that is overbearing. It gets sick and tired and fights back by generating an inflammatory response, which in turn makes you feel tired, bloated, foggy, and the list goes on.

By removing dairy from your diet you give your digestive system a break, so that when it's re-introduced into your diet it doesn't have the same negative effect on your gut. It's like giving yourself a two weeks' vacation. Before you go on vacation you feel exhausted, inefficient and can't stand any more work or projects. While on vacation, you feel relaxed and happy and forget about all your work troubles. When you go back to work you are fresh and energized, eager to face and take over any workload. This energy stays with you for a while, until your energy tank gets depleted again and a new cycle begins.

The same thing happens to your gut. Over time, it's energy and ability to efficiently digest and extract nutrients from the food ingested gets depleted as a result of the eroding effects of certain foods and environment.   By giving your gut a break from foods known to irritate and stress the digestive tract you reignite your gut's health and ability to better digest food.

Don't get me wrong, dairy is not completely evil. I love cheese and I still have it in moderation (especially goat cheese, which is known to be easier to digest). But, since our body can get overloaded with dairy and as we age we make fewer enzymes that help digest the protein in it, we need to give our body time to replenish.

At the end of the elimination period, it's up to you to determine if dairy is indeed a problem for you and you might even choose to eliminate it for a longer period of time or for good. Some people do well with dairy, while others struggle with digestive distress and sinus problems as a result. Listen to your body and determine what's best for you. At the end of the day, your body is your best doctor.

Foods to Avoid

- ❀ Milk in any form

- ❀ Cheese (any type)

- ❀ Yogurt

- ❀ Kefir

- ❀ Butter

- ❀ Buttermilk

- ❀ Casein containing foods

- ❀ Whey containing foods and whey protein

- ❀ Food alternatives to dairy

- ❀ Tofu

- ❀ Alternative cheese cream spread ("Tofutti: Better than cheese cream")

- ❀ Almond cheese

- ❀ Nutritional yeast (good for imitating cheese flavor in vegan dishes)

- ❀ Nut butter (cashews and almonds make great butter that can be used instead of cheese in gluten-free lasagna or other recipes calling for cheese)

Sugar

The biggest enemy to your Gut's health is refined sugar. Any white sugars and high fructose corn syrup should be completely avoided.

In my opinion, and more than likely that of other holistic health addicts like me, refined sugar is a form of poison, a drug made legal by the Food Industry only to get us hooked on all the unhealthy packaged food found at every corner.

According to research published in the NY Times, sugar is habit forming and creates addiction just as much as cocaine and nicotine, producing the same symptoms reported by substance abuse and dependence. These are craving, tolerance, and withdrawal. Based on studies performed on rats, sugar is preferred over cocaine as it gives a more pleasurable high. [11]

As scary as this sounds, we might not realize the effect sugar has on us until we steer free from consuming it. That's when we start realizing how addicted we are.

Aside from the addicting effect sugar has on us, it also contributes to the deterioration of the gut flora, leaving us susceptible to gastrointestinal distress, infections, and mood disorders.

Unfriendly bacteria, such as candida, feeds on sugar, so the more sugar we eat the more unfriendly bacteria develops to eat away our good

---

11 (Dinicolantonio and Lucan)

friends. The healthy balance between good versus bad bacteria is negatively impacted and that's the first step to an unhealthy and unbalanced Gut. When our Gut is out of balance our whole self is out of balance, opening the door for various diseases.

Just like money is the root of all evil, I say, sugar is the evil of all health!

What to Avoid

❁ White, refined sugar

❁ High fructose corn syrup

❁ Any store bought baked goods (as they are full of unhealthy fats and sugars)

❁ Protein bars made with sugar or high corn syrup

❁ Candies

❁ Packaged foods containing sugar

In order to correctly implement this step in the process, you need to get in the habit of reading labels. I can't stress that enough, but you will notice that there are lots of hidden sources of sugar in almost all packaged food you buy. The best way to avoid the hidden sugars is to stay away from the middle section isles of your conventional grocery store.

Common Names for Sugar You Should be on the Lookout For

- ❖ Glucose
- ❖ Fructose
- ❖ Sucrose
- ❖ High Fructose Corn Syrup (or HFCS)
- ❖ Molasses
- ❖ Evaporated Cane Sugar/Juice
- ❖ Refiner's Syrup
- ❖ Corn Syrup
- ❖ Dextrose
- ❖ Dextrin
- ❖ Ethyl Matlol
- ❖ Maltodextrin
- ❖ Matlose
- ❖ Barley Malt
- ❖ Sucanat

Alternatives to Sugar [12]

In order to make the transition smoother and reduce cravings I recommend the following substitutes for sugar:

❋ Agave syrup (known to be low on the glycemic index scale, thus it doesn't create the same spike in glucose as sugar does)

❋ Coconut sugar

❋ Honey in moderation

❋ Maple syrup in moderation

❋ Medjool dates paste (blended dry dates are a natural way of sweetening your deserts)

❋ Stevia (a natural sweetener that has zero calories; tends to taste way too sweet, so use lower quantities)

12 © Integrative Nutrition Inc.(used with permission)

Tips for Reducing Cravings

Add naturally sweet vegetables to your diet

Such as butternut squash, sweet potatoes, carrots, parsley root, and celery root. This will reduce your need and craving of eating sweets, as your body already gets what it needs.

Eat fresh fruits as dessert

Opt for berries when available, as they don't have a lot of naturally occurring sugars and are a great source of antioxidants. It's a win-win!

Eat more protein.

Sometimes sweet cravings are a sign that you are not consuming enough protein. Your body mistakenly craves sweets, when in fact it needs more protein. By simply adding more protein to your diet your sweet cravings will dissipate.

Drink plenty of water

Sometimes your craving could occur from thirst without realizing it.

Practice self-care

So you satisfy your needs on a deeper level. Many times your cravings for food are a result of lack of love or self-care. This is something I will cover more in Step 2 of the program.

As far as sugar goes, although I recommend removing it from your diet for at least 2 weeks, I highly recommend removing refined sugar and especially high fructose corn sugar for good. If you have to use sugar down the road, past the completion of this program, try to use non-refined options, such as unrefined cane sugar or in the raw turbinado sugar. Although I suggest you use the alternatives to sugar mentioned above as a way of living and use it in moderation.

Get in the habit of making your own home-cooked desserts so you have control over the amount and type of sweetener used.

My client Geta used to be hooked on sweets. Once she started eating some (especially cookies) she would have a hard time stopping. Every time she did that she had to deal with all kinds of gastrointestinal issues to the point where she lost hope. When she started working with me, she complained about feeling tired all the time and, of course, about IBS related issues. She followed my program and after only one month she reported major improvements in her energy, weight and best of all – she took control of her cravings. In her own words, she said, "I can't believe that I don't crave sweets anymore. I don't even think of it. That's never happened to me." All because she started eating whole foods that provided all the nutrients her body craved. She ate from all the food groups and satisfied all the 6 tastes according to the Ayuverdic medicine: salty, sweet, sour, pungent, bitter and astringent.

When you give your body what it needs to stay balanced, your cravings dissipate. Your plate is balanced and so are you. This is the state you need to aim for when choosing healthy eating and balanced living. This is the lifestyle I promote and the ultimate goal of this program.

Final thoughts on the elimination stage

You won't have to give up all of the ingredients mentioned in this stage of the process for the rest of your life. Think of it as a cleanse that will refresh your entire body giving you more energy for better assimilation of nutrients, better digestion and most of all an overall feeling of wellbeing and clarity.

You will feel like you just came out of a trance in which you were just going with the flow without being totally awake, without being able to enjoy life and move on with clarity and energy. You will be surprised by how much your energy will improve and how good life could feel if you feed your body foods that actually nurture and heal you and not the other way around!

The purpose of this stage is to give your digestive system a break from the invading effects of some of the harder to digest foods that could be or not a problem for you personally. Additionally, eliminating these foods from your diet for a certain period of time will help you identify if any of them could represent potential food sensitivity when reintroduced back into your diet.

However, please don't mistake food sensitivity for food allergy! These two have very different reactions and an allergy could be life threatening. Food sensitivities typically occur in people with more sensitive digestive systems, when our body has a harder time digesting that particular food and it needs time away from it in order to heal and learn to better deal with it. If you think you may have a food allergy, please see your doctor.

Possible Signs of Food Sensitivity

Here are some of the symptoms that could indicate that your body has a harder time digesting a certain food group and might need more time away from it:

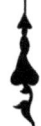

- Headaches

- Foggy brain

- Fatigue

- Tummy aches

- Moodiness

- Sinus congestion (typical for dairy sensitivity and even gluten)

- Lack of concentration

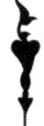

If you notice any of these symptoms after the reintroduction of a food group, chances are that you might not be in good terms with that food group and you would be better off giving yourself more time away from it. Your body might need more time to desensitize itself from it. But, rest assured, once you finished implementing the next action steps for a healthier Gut, and feel good about the way you eat and feel, you can reintroduce that food group again. Chances are, your Gut is now functioning and digesting better and you will not have a problem enjoying your favorite food once more.

One piece of advice, though, is to not exaggerate consuming that food group, so you don't over-saturate your gut with it and trigger sensitivity symptoms again.

I myself discovered I have a sensitivity to gluten and dairy for instance. And after a long time of not consuming gluten and dairy I now went back to consuming them occasionally, but not relying on them daily. For instance, if I go to a nice restaurant where they have something yummy with gluten or cheese I will willingly indulge myself every here and there, knowing that I will not consume that again for at least several days after. It's *Joshua's 90-10 Diet*[13] – eat right most of the time and indulge yourself once in a while. I religiously apply this in every aspect of my life and I encourage you to try it! It gives you the confidence that you are in control. And when you live your life like this, you truly are!

The Reintroduction Stage

After the elimination period, slowly reintroduce one food group at a time into your diet and make note of any changes you might experience. I highly recommend keeping a food journal during both the elimination and reintroduction stage (see food journal pages at the end of the book for easy tracking). If, for instance, when gluten was reintroduced to your system your symptoms came back, chances are gluten might be a problem for you and you should avoid it for a longer period of time or consume it only occasionally. Either way, talk to your doctor about your symptoms to rule out a more serious condition. Follow the same steps for dairy and sugar as well.

I recommend that you give yourself 2 days of experimenting with the reintroduction of each food group, so you can notice any possible symptoms or side effects as a result of the consumption of the respective food.

---

13 ©2008 Integrative Nutrition Inc. (used with permission)

Start with gluten or dairy, whatever you missed most, and wait 2 days before you add in the next food group. If your body reacts negatively, it will do so within 2 days. If no side effects were noticed move on to the second food group.

Now, if you are one of the lucky ones and none of the foods eliminated seem to trigger any pain point then you are all set. Your body needed some time to refresh and now it's functioning even better. You couldn't be in a better place than this. Aside from cleansing your body and feeling great, you gained more energy and you even lost a few pounds! Win-win!

As a rule of thumb, though, for keeping up with healthy eating – just like you will see in the section to follow – I recommend that if you choose to consume gluten, you opt for whole grain as often as possible (whole wheat, spelt, and the likes). As far as dairy goes, aim for goat-based cheeses and yogurts when possible, as they are easier to digest and less likely to trigger sensitivity related symptoms.

Reduce Toxic Load (Eat Organic and Local)

The second stage in cleaning out your plate is focused on reducing toxic load.

Pesticides, GMOs (genetically modified organisms) and any other chemicals used in harvesting crops and in overly-processed foods should be avoided to the best of our ability. Long-term consumption of foods containing these harmful ingredients could add to the toxic load of our body. As a result, our immunity gets compromised, we get tired easier, we experience fogginess, loss of energy and thus we have a harder time fighting infections and digesting food.

More so, studies looking at the connection between pesticide use and cancer have shown a positive relationship between exposure to pesticides and the development of some cancers, particularly in children.[14] With the increased use of pesticides in the US, no wonder we live in a society where cancer in all forms has become more and more common.

The best way to minimize toxic load is to eat organic whenever possible and opt for local and seasonal produce when organic is out of reach due to price or availability.

Actually, when you eat with the season you tend to eat more locally-grown produce, which is a lot healthier than eating produce that has been grown far away and went through long shipments and many hands until it reached your table. The more hands and time involved until it reaches your table, the less nutrient dense your food is.

So, when you can, go for locally-grown produce and adjust your eating habits and menu based on what's fresh and in season. Chances are the produce that's in season and locally grown is cheaper as well. What better reason to keep your eyes open for local and seasonal produce?

The second most important way of minimizing toxic load is to cut down on overly-processed foods, such as packaged goods found in the middle sections of the conventional supermarkets. You know which

---

14 (Bassil, Vakil and Sanborn)

ones they are. The ones that have a long shelf life and are filled with hydrogenated oils, sugars and tons of preservatives and ingredients you can't pronounce.

Go to http://healthyzesty.com/3-day-healthy-zesty-jumpstart-menu to download your FREE copy.

HEAL YOUR GUT - ACTION STEP 2

Eat Whole

Eating whole means eating your food in its most natural state. Eating as nature intended! This way, you know exactly what it is that you put into your body, without any hidden and possibly harmful ingredients.

The best way to stay away from overly-processed foods and embrace a healthy diet is to eat whole! And I don't mean shopping only at Whole Foods (although I must admit that's one of my guilty pleasures), but eating whole, unrefined and unprocessed foods. The more refined food is, the less nutrient dense it gets and the more it starves your cells of important nutrients, which ultimately affects your health and weight. As if they aren't bad enough already, refined foods accentuate your cravings! The more refined food you eat, the more sugar and carbs you crave.

What do you think is the opposite of nutrient-dense foods? Calorie-dense foods! Which means you can eat a lot more of the nutrient-dense foods without adding to your waistline, whereas the calorie-dense foods produce a sudden spike in glucose, which promotes weight gain. So, I don't know about you, but I'll go for the nutrient-dense foods. Not only does it keep my weight and cravings in check, but I know it nurtures my body at a cellular level, which is what drives health.

Eating whole is a practice you should adopt for the rest of your life and not for just a few weeks. This is actually what a healthy-zesty diet looks like. But this is not one of those fad diets that promise to make us look and feel better. We all know how that goes. We get excited at the inception of each new diet, hoping for a miracle, only to find ourselves deprived and disappointed a couple of weeks later (if we can make it that far). That's why they are just that: A Diet! We tend to fall off that diet just a few weeks later, landing back where we started or worse, developing mood swings and uncontrollable cravings. This is typically a normal reaction in the case of an unbalanced diet, which some of the fad diets promote. However, eating whole allows us to eat the entire spectrum of the food plate, but in a whole form and without certain ingredients listed in Step 1 for a limited period of time. When eating whole you tend to eat more fruits and vegetables and your body gets all nutrients it needs to thrive, thus cravings are diminished. And this to me is not a restrictive diet, but a healthy way of eating and living.

When choosing a diet you have to choose one you can stick to long term. One that is in line with your lifestyle and promotes balanced living and long-term health benefits. One that can become a Lifestyle! And that's what a healthy-zesty diet is supposed to be – a Lifestyle!

The secret to following a healthy-zesty diet consists of crowding out[15] the bad stuff and adding in more of the good stuff.

---

15 © 2007 Integrative Nutrition Inc. (used with permission)

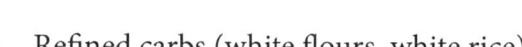

What to Crowd Out

- Refined carbs (white flours, white rice)

- Refined sugars (white sugar, high fructose corn syrup)

- Overly-processed foods (packaged food and anything that requires multiple refining processes before it ends on the shelf)

- Trans fats (check labels for partially hydrogenated oil, or trans fats)

- Artificial sweeteners and food coloring

- Anything hard to pronounce

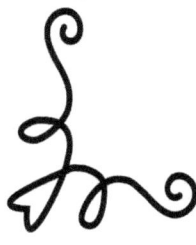
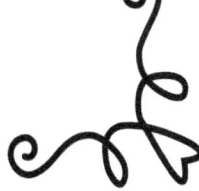

What to Add In

- ❁ Vegetables (the more the merrier)

- ❁ Leafy greens (the greener the better)

- ❁ Fruits (especially berries, as they are rich in anti-oxidants and low in sugars)

- ❁ Whole grains (gluten-free oats, brown rice, quinoa, millet, buckwheat and whole wheat when gluten is not an issue)

- ❁ Fish (wild fish, such as salmon, sardines, and Alaskan wild cod)

- ❁ Meats (preferably organic poultry and lean meats)

- ❁ Legumes (beans, chickpeas, peas)

- ❁ Nuts

- ❁ Olive oil

- ❁ Tea

- ❁ Spices (turmeric, ginger, garlic and cinnamon have known anti-inflammatory properties)

Sounds easy as pie, right? It's really no brainer. It only takes a little bit of time and coordination to start incorporating this diet into your lifestyle and reaping the health benefits it brings. I encourage you to experiment with it and get into the habit of reading labels. By the end of the program, you might decide that you don't need any meat, other than just fish and (which is what I did). Or you could decide to drop dairy altogether or eat only goat-based dairy. Whatever works for you and fits your lifestyle and body type. That's what I love about a truly healthy diet. It gives you so many options to choose from without feeling deprived. You will be surprised by how much your energy and outlook on life will change once you adopt a healthy diet, even if the only thing you do is increase the intake of fruits and vegetables or cut down on refined and processed foods. I know it made a tremendous difference in my life and that of my family.

I remember before I changed my diet and lifestyle I used to eat whatever was handy, without really thinking of health consequences or the content of what I was consuming. Not to mention that reading labels was not on my mind. I didn't see the connection between what I ate and how I felt. But once I started taking small steps toward changing my diet and implemented these changes I am sharing with you in this book, my awareness around health, nutrition and self-care became so heightened that it completely changed the way I look at food.

Once you start eating whole foods, your cravings will disappear and you'll naturally make better choices when eating out or snacking. And trust me, you'll feel so good and energized that you won't want to throw that down the drain for the sake of a sugary and overly-processed treat that will only make you feel tired and moody soon after consuming it.

Don't get me wrong, nobody is expecting you to eat a perfectly healthy diet 24/7. No way! Even I know that's impossible. But you need to have a reference point – an indicator of what a healthy diet means to you – which is what will help you take control over what you put into your body most of the time. Without a reference point, you have no goal, no final destination; no way of knowing if you are on the right path or not. So aiming for a healthy-zesty diet should be your final goal, but making a conscious decision to spoil yourself once in a while with something that is out of the norm is perfectly fine.

Remember *Joshua's 90-10 Diet*[16] (or you can even make it 80/20 if it sounds more reasonable to you)? That's what this is about – eating right most of the time but allowing yourself the liberty to be bad and indulge yourself every now and then. It is perfectly okay and I strongly encourage this type of attitude. This is going to give you a sense of satisfaction you won't get otherwise if you had no rules around your way of eating. But in this case, you are in control. You decide when you want to go bad and you enjoy that moment to its fullest.

I personally like to do something different on Friday nights or Saturdays, for instance. We either go out and I eat something more indulging than usual, or I personally bake a dessert (although I usually make it with healthier ingredients than the ones I would get with a commercially bought dessert, which is so much more satisfying). So, how are you going to indulge yourself? What's going to be your special treat and reward for being good to your body?

---

16 ©2008 Integrative Nutrition Inc. (used with permission)

HEAL YOUR GUT - ACTION STEP 3

Hydrate

D rink plenty of water. I really can't stress enough the importance of water in our life, and more so for a healthy gut.

Water is indeed the foundation of life. We are made of 75% water and our brain alone is 85% water. We can live up to 3 weeks without food (Mahatma Gandhi survived 21 days completely without food), but some say we can't go more than a week without water. That alone is proof of the importance of water for proper functioning.

Drinking enough water allows your body to better flush out toxins, an important process for weight loss and overall wellbeing. Additionally, lack of water can throw off the balance between good versus bad intestinal bacteria, leading to inflammation and gut-related issues (including bloating and constipation).

How Much Water Do You Need?

How much water you need depends on your body type, climate, activity level, age, and diet. But as a general rule of thumb, you should be consuming in average about 8 glasses of water a day, or the equivalent of 2 liters of water if you weigh around 135 pounds. More water might be needed if you have a larger body structure and exercise more frequently.

A back of the envelope calculation for determining the quantity of water needed based only on weight is to divide your weight in pounds by 2, which gives you the quantity of recommended water consumption in ounces.

Side Effects of Too Little Water [17]

If you don't consume enough water your body could experience the following side effects:

- ❋ Headaches

- ❋ Hunger (many times when you think you are hungry you are actually thirsty, so try to drink more water when you experience sudden hunger)

- ❋ Sugar cravings

- ❋ Fatigue

- ❋ Foggy thinking

17 © Integrative Nutrition Inc.(used with permission)

Beware of Dehydrating Drinks

Certain drinks you consume during the day could cause dehydration, thus requiring that you up the quantity of water consumed.

Coffee, black teas, soda, energy drinks and alcohol, although contain some water, are not hydrating due to the dehydrating agents found in caffeine, alcohol, and other ingredients.

Go to www.healthyzesty.com/3-day-healthy-zesty-jumpstart-menu to download your 3-day menu!

Rebalance Intestinal Flora

As I mentioned in the beginning of this chapter, achieving an optimal balance of good versus bad intestinal bacteria is key to your gut health. An unbalanced gut opens the door to digestive distress, infections and overall inflammation generated ailments.

The collection of intestinal flora in your gut, known as microbiota, is responsible for how you feel as it has a direct impact on your immune function, nutrient assimilation, infections, bowel movements, GI health and overall mood and energy. It is even thought that an unbalanced gut flora could lead to food allergies and sensitivities.

Therefore, it's important that you maintain the optimal 85/15 balance between good versus bad bacteria in your gut. For that, you need to promote and nourish friendly bacteria.

How to Promote Friendly Bacteria (think probiotics)

A well-balanced Gut helps us fully digest food, properly absorb nutrients from food, and keeps infections and viruses at bay. For that, we need to increase the intake of beneficial bacteria, known as probiotic, through our diet or/and probiotic supplements (always check with your doctor before starting a new supplement regimen).

Dr. Derrick M. DeSilva, a highly-respected Integrative Medicine physician, used to say, "If you don't love someone in your family, you should not put them on a probiotic supplement." That for me did the trick. Everybody in my family takes a probiotic supplement now. Based on my own experience, probiotic supplements are essential for a healthy immune system and a well-balanced gut. For my family and me, this is a must, no matter how much probiotic-rich food we consume.

Probiotic Supplements

There is a vast variety of available probiotics out there, but not all are created equal, so please look for the ones that have more strains of microorganisms and 5 billion or more CFU (colony forming units). This is just a suggestion and depending on your own situation you may or may not need a probiotic supplement, although I am a big believer in the benefits of probiotics. Always check with your doctor before starting a new supplement regimen.

These are the main species and strains of probiotics:

❖ Lactobacillus Species: acidophilus, spo-rogenes, salivarius, casei, kefir, bulgaricus (found predominantly in the small intestine)

❖ Bifidobacterium Species: bifidum, longum, infantus (found predominantly in the large intestine)

❖ S. thermophiles

❖ Saccharomyces boulardii

Probiotic Rich Food

Aside from considering adding a potent probiotic supplement to your daily routine, you should focus on consuming more of the following foods, rich in friendly bacteria:

❖ Fermented foods, such as vegetables in brine (e.g. sauerkraut, pickles)

❖ Kefir

❖ Yogurt (unsweetened)

❖ Umeboshi (pickled ume fruits found in Japan, translated into English as "Japanese salt plums)

❖ Miso soup

❖ Tempeh

❖ Kimchi (traditional fermented Korean side

dish made of vegetables, mainly cabbage with a variety of seasonings

❀ Kombucha tea/drink (a type of fermented tea you can find typically in health stores)

How to Nourish Friendly Bacteria (think prebiotics)

Friendly bacteria thrives in your colon and digestive tract with the help of prebiotics. Prebiotics are actually non-digestible dietary fibers and can be found in some probiotic supplements under the name of inulin, but they are also present in certain plants, as you will see below.

Now that your gut is populated with good bacteria, thanks to the pro-biotic you are taking, it is important to properly feed the intestinal flora and keep it at healthy levels. You can do this by taking a prebiotic sup-plement (such as inulin or oligofructose) and/or eating more prebiotic rich foods, such as:

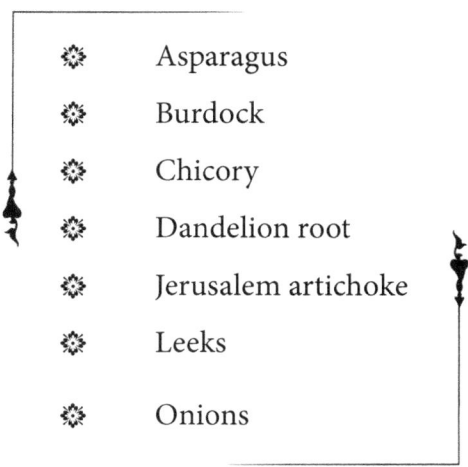

❀ Asparagus

❀ Burdock

❀ Chicory

❀ Dandelion root

❀ Jerusalem artichoke

❀ Leeks

❀ Onions

So, next time you need to give your Gut a hand at keeping your gut friends happy, add some more of these plants to your diet.

HEAL YOUR GUT - ACTION STEP 5

Support Your Digestion

with Digestive Enzymes and Bitters

This section focuses on making things easier on your digestive system so it doesn't work as hard and properly assimilates the nutrients in the deliciously healthy food you are now eating.

Digestive enzymes aid in the digestion and assimilation of your food, so it passes through the entire digestive tract without delay and is efficiently converted into waste and promptly eliminated.

If you tend to have a slower digestion I suggest you try a naturally derived digestive enzyme supplement once you vetted this with your doctor. You can find such supplements at Whole Foods or other health stores.

I suggest you take one supplement with each meal in the first 2 weeks while on the elimination diet, and after that only take it with the heaviest meal of the day (typically with dinner, or dinner and lunch if you feel the need to).

I personally only take a digestive enzyme supplement when I travel and eat out a lot, although, I used to take one with every meal in the first months of my recovery.

The most natural and delicious way of boosting your digestion is through actual food, though. The following foods and herbs are known to aid digestion and soothe inflammation:

❈ Papaya – rich in digestive enzymes. Helps break down lactose.

❈ Beets – stimulate the release of bile, thus helping break down fats. It is good in liver detoxification cures.

❈ Dandelion (greens or tea) – stimulates the gall-bladder, liver, and pancreas to release bile and digestive enzymes. Good cleansing agent and detoxifier.

❈ Ginger – soothes inflammation of the gut, calms down nausea and helps digestion.

You can use all or any of these foods in your morning smoothie for stimulating your digestive juices and prepping you for a glorious day! Go ahead and experiment with any of these and reap the benefits of better digestion.

HEAL YOUR GUT - ACTION STEP 6

Get Cooking

When it comes to eating healthy, whole and clean, which is what the healthy-zesty diet is all about, the best way to stay on course is to get cooking. Experimenting with home-cooked meals is not only healthier but cheaper and more satisfying. There is a special connection, an energy we create with the food we cook ourselves, which makes it more nutritious and fulfilling. Plus, we tend to eat less when we eat at home, an added benefit if you are one of those people who keep an eye on the scale.

Like Julia Child said - "*You don't have to cook fancy or complicated masterpieces – just good food from fresh ingredients*".

Keep it simple and don't stress out. Always remember the why behind your actions so you keep yourself motivated on the path to healthy eating and happy living!

Benefits of Practicing Home Cooking

Relaxes your mind.

By engaging in cooking – especially when following a recipe or a certain sequence of steps – your mind stops wandering and is more present in the moment, similar to meditating. You are fully ingrained into the cooking process, thus more self-aware, and all your negative thoughts or worries dissipate. Even if it's just for a while. It's like being engaged in the creation of a piece of art. It is both relaxing and satisfying (not only for you but for your dear ones as well, especially when they savor your piece of art).

Healing Energy.

Your food carries the energy of the person who cooked it, the place it was cooked in and of course the ingredients used. If you eat in a restaurant where there is a lot of agitation in the kitchen and food is being handled with anger or discontent, all that energy will be transmitted to your food and, later on, to you. Have you ever wonder why you felt tired or you got indigestion after you went out to a certain restaurant for dinner? There is a connection. It is the energy of food, which could be positive or negative. Unless, of course, the food was contaminated with some unwanted bacteria.

On the other hand, when you cook your food with love, curiosity and calm your food will have healing effects over you and your family. It's full of good vibes, full of positive energy! And it tastes better when it's cooked with love! That's why I always add Vitamin L® (from Love) as an ingredient to any of my recipes! And you should, too! But if you are mad and angry when cooking, I suggest you calm down before you immerse yourself into cooking, so you don't poison yourself or others! Or you should just eat out; sometimes that's better when cooking feels like an unpleasant chore that will only add more stress to you. When you engage yourself in cooking, you should do so with curiosity and never with anger, especially if cooking is a new territory for you. You might even discover you like it.

Control over quality and quantity of ingredients.

You never know what goes into the food you eat in a restaurant or how many hands your food went through before it reached your table. Instead, when you cook you know exactly what goes into your food and think twice before you add something that doesn't sound as healthy. You have a better chance of eating food made from fresh ingredients and you know how to practice portion control, without feeling sorry that the leftovers will go down the drain, just like your money. Instead, the food you cooked can be saved for enjoying the next day, saving you the trouble of spending more time in the kitchen.

Cook once - eat twice.

When cooking at home, get into the habit of cooking a bigger meal, so you can enjoy same food without extra effort the next day as well. You can do this in 2 ways:

Double the portion of your dinner dish, such that you enjoy an encore the next day for dinner as well. Or better yet, make a soup once a week and enjoy it up to 3 days. When you eat soup with dinner you can easily have a light salad as a second dish without feeling deprived.

Use leftovers in a different recipe next day for lunch or breakfast. For instance, if you made brown rice with fish and vegetables the night before, use the extra rice for a breakfast porridge or for lunch, by adding some veggies and tofu or chicken to it.

Helps you stick to a healthy diet.

We all know that most restaurants tend to use way too much salt, sugar, refined carbs or unhealthy fats in order to make their food more appealing. Just like we know that we should reduce the consumption of such ingredients. So how can you do that? By eating more home-cooked meals. This way, you know exactly what goes on your plate and into your belly. Not to mention that you won't have to constantly go back and forth when checking the menu, talking yourself into giving in to your temptations. We all know it's harder to fight temptation than to avoid it. When you eat home, there is no temptation. What you cook is what you get. But if the options are there, then watch out will powers!

But don't get me wrong – I am not saying you should not eat out. No way! You should actually indulge yourself to dining out a couple of times a week (or even more if need be, but please stay away from fast food restaurants!). And when you do go out, try to make that feel special. The idea is to change the balance between eating in and eating out, by leaning toward eating in more often than eating out. Say you use to eat out five days out of seven. Start by going out four days out of seven at first and keep making your way to more home-cooked days than restaurant days. At the end of the day, eating out needs to be the exception, not the rule. Eating out should be something we do in order to spoil ourselves and even relax by changing the scenery and why not, menu. And what's best is that aside from helping you stick to a cleaner, healthier diet, it will also make you enjoy more of those little things, like going out, instead of taking them for granted.

Have you ever wondered why the restaurant business, especially fast food, is such a blooming business in America? Because people here do eat out a lot, unlike other parts of the world. For that reason, America has the biggest obesity rate.

Brings family and friends together.

This is, by far, my favorite part of eating in! Picture those old movies where the entire family gathers around the table eager to discover the yummy home-cooked dishes. Everybody is happily talking about their day and a special connection is being re-created. It is, really, the only time when everybody gets to sit together and focus on the same masterpiece: mom's dinner (or dad's dinner!). This is an image we should all attempt to recreate in our homes. It is how it used to be and what kept families united. When you think of it, obesity, divorce, depression, ADHD, autism or any other behavior-related diseases were not as prevalent as they are in today's society. I know things changed, we evolved and have higher expectations. And we should. But wouldn't you agree that we should have higher expectations for the quality of our food, for the way food is supposed to make us feel?

You probably wonder what does food have to do with how you feel. Well, a lot! If you feel exhausted all the time and foggy, don't you think that's a direct result of what you fuel your body with every day? Just like a car – when you load it with high octane gas it runs smoother and without hiccups. And it's just a car, not a living being. Now imagine how big of an impact real, clean food could have on your energy.

You are busy, I understand. You are always chasing time like there is no tomorrow and you must wonder when in the world will you have time to actually cook. It might seem hard at first, but believe me, once you've mastered the planning of it everything becomes routine and takes less time than going out to pick up dinner. You just need to plan in advance and voila! Your stress disappears and your food gets cleaner!

I don't know about you, but nothing gives me more pleasure than spending time with friends. And there is nothing more satisfying than sharing a nice dinner with my friends and collecting compliments for a well done, delicious dinner. I know it takes a bit more effort to prepare dinner for a big gathering, but the reward is that much bigger. An event like this satisfies the need for *Primary Food*[18] and *Secondary Food*[19].

The *Primary Food*[18] is what nurtures you on the inside (such as the need to socialize, to feel appreciated, to connect with others and escape the routine). And getting together with friends, with or without dinner, does just that.

The *Secondary Food*[19], on the other hand, is the food we eat; what we need to survive. And according to my teacher, Joshua Rosenthal from the Institute for Integrative Nutrition®, food is secondary because when your *Primary Food*[18] is satisfied, your life actually feeds you at a deeper level and food becomes less important, it becomes secondary. This is something I will be talking more about in the pages to follow, as reaching a balance between the two aspects – *Primary Food*[18] and *Secondary Food*[19] – is what we all should be aiming for in order to feel healthy and zesty.

---

18 ©2005 Integrative Nutrition Inc. (used with permission)
19 ©2005 Integrative Nutrition Inc. (used with permission)

The Healthy-Zesty Meal Planning

By now you must have gotten the idea behind the Healthy Zesty diet and the role it plays in keeping your gut balanced and leading a Healthy Zesty life. Easy as pie, right?

Well, easier said than done, you may think. But please don't fret; I am here to your rescue. My Healthy Zesty meal planning tips will make it easier for you to actually go do it and not just read it. The tips below will help you get crystal clear on your task and how you can actually implement all these changes into your life, so you can truly enjoy the benefits of a Healthy Zesty diet and feel and look your best!

The secret to keeping up with a healthy eating regimen is planning. Without it, you'll find yourself running like a chicken without head come Monday evening when everybody gathers home from a long day of work or school.

How can you avoid this? Plan ahead!

Meal Planning Tips

The tips below will help you successfully implement the steps for improving your gut health and boosting your energy, without feeling frustrated or deprived.

1. Plan your week ahead on Sunday

Set aside 30 minutes on Sunday morning to brainstorm on what your week ahead will look like as far as planned events and meals.

Write down the days you'll be eating home and what you are planning to have for dinner and even lunch on those days. Use the shopping lists provided at the end of this section when making decisions around your menu or download my 3-Day Healthy Zesty Jumpstart Menu for complete menu with recipes developed specifically to reset your gut for better digestion and improved energy.

> Go to http://healthyzesty.com/3-day-healthy-zesty-jumpstart-menu to download your FREE copy.

2. Look for recipes

Dust off your old recipe books, search online or go to my website (www. healthyzesty.com) to pick the recipes for the coming week. Look for gluten-free, dairy-free recipes, especially during the first 2 weeks while on the elimination diet. The recipes included in the 3-Day Healthy Zesty Jumpstart Menu are all gluten-free and dairy-free, so I suggest you start there, as they were specifically developed for this program.

3. Make your shopping list

Once you decided what recipes to try, make a list with the ingredients you need. Check off the ones you already have in your fridge or pantry.

Use the lists provided at the end of this section when choosing the ingredients for your recipes. Even if the recipe calls for something not on this list, don't be afraid to play and make your own healthy substitutions. You'll soon become a master at this.

4. *Tour the Food Store*

Next stop is your local food store. Plan on doing your shopping on Sunday afternoon, or evening for at least 3 days, so you don't waste more time on your way home from work. Instead, you'll use that time for preparing a delicious and healthy dinner.

When at a grocery store, steer away from the middle aisle section, as that is typically packed with unhealthy options, such as overly processed foods that usually come in a box. Instead, focus on the side sections, typically dedicated to fresh produce, where you'll find natural, whole produce, and fresh meats and dairies (go for dairy free milk options though).

5.*Make double batches*

Remember my earlier tip - cook once, eat twice? When making a recipe plan on doubling the ingredients, such that you can eat the same meal for 2 days. Or, if eating the same dinner is not appealing to you, get in the habit of using dinner leftovers for a makeover lunch.

6. *Prep your lunch and dinner the night before*

Depending on what you've planned for next day's dinner, determine if there is any prepping activity that can be done the night before. For example:

* ❁ Chop your veggies and place them in the fridge until next day when ready to cook them or assemble them into a nice salad.

❁ Steam the brown rice (that usually takes longer to make, so it's helpful to cook it ahead of time). You could choose to only pre-cook it and put it back in the rice cooker for just 15 minutes the next day. Or you can just warm it up in the microwave the next day if completely cooked already. Just remember to add a tablespoon of water over it and loosely cover it with a lid or plastic foil.

❁ Season the fish, tofu or meat the night before and lace them into a Ziploc bag. You could also let them marinade overnight, which will make them that much tastier.

❁ Pack your lunch and place it in the fridge until next morning.

7. The great old salad

When everything else fails, the great old salad comes to the rescue!

When you ran out of ideas for dinner, or you just didn't have time to plan for it, just reach for the great old salad. You could never go wrong there.

Here are some tips for keeping your salad always fresh, nutritious and tasty:

❁ Always make your own dressing. Just mix lemon juice, olive oil, salt and pepper and optionally a teaspoon of agave nectar when looking for a slightly sweet taste in your dressing. You could even blend in some berries or avocado, for variety in texture and flavor.

❀ Pack your fridge with 2 different types of salads so you can alternate or even mix (go for dark green options when available, such as baby spinach, kale, Swiss chard, arugula, romaine).

❀ Experiment with fruits. Add fruits to your salad for a slightly sweet kick that will also make it more appealing to your kids (it will definitely make it more appealing to you too). Every time you make a salad try a new fruit, whatever you have in the fridge that day. It could be raspberries, strawberries, apples, pears, grapes, mangoes, pineapple, etc. Be creative!

❀ Keep a variety of nuts handy to add to your salad for added protein and consistency (walnuts, sliced almonds, pine nuts, pecans).

❀ Don't be afraid of seeds. Hemp seeds and chia seeds, for instance, are super-foods that could nicely complement your salad when you are looking for a more potent salad.

❀ Use dried fruits to add sweetness and variety to your salad.

❀ Add crunchiness to your salad by using: onions, celery, shredded carrots, radicchio, peppers, pomegranate seeds or even some iceberg lettuce.

❁ Add flavor with toppings. Top your salad with fresh spices and greens, such as cilantro, parsley, dill, basil.

❁ Add protein. Use your favorite protein, for a complete meal. Go for organic or grass-fed meats when possible, wild fish, beans, tofu, hummus, nuts.

❁ Get creative. Don't be afraid to experiment with different veggies, fruits, and toppings whenever you make a salad. Just base your salad on the ingredients you have in the fridge that day.

8. Keep snacks handy

Always have healthy snacks alternatives in your bag, pantry, or fridge. Nuts of all kinds are a good option, as you could carry them with you anywhere. Aside from being convenient, they are packed with healthy fats and proteins that give you energy, keeping the hunger in check.

9. Mindful eating

Last, but not least, sit down for a mindful dinner. Give yourself some credit for your hard work and for making your dinner as healthy and tasty as possible. Slow down and chew completely and mindfully. Notice the medley of flavors in your mouth and be grateful for it.

To make it even more special you can light a candle and make sure you turn off your TV or other distractions. My family and I have a very strict ritual around dinner: cell phones away, TV off, relaxing music on! And the rest is just conversation around the food and the good things that happened that day. Nothing negative or disturbing around the dinner table!

10. *Healthy Zesty Approved Shopping List*

When grocery shopping and cooking, try to use as many ingredients from the first two tables, as those are the ones making the biggest impact on your overall health. Vegetables and leafy greens are packed with anti-oxidants and polyphenols, known to protect against cancers and promote healthy cells.

Additionally, get in the habit of using anti-inflammatory herbs in your cooking. Aside from enhancing flavor, they have undeniable health benefits. You can never have too many spices and herbs, except of course for the chili pepper and other overly spicy herbs (although spicy food helps with speeding up your metabolism).

Leafy Greens	
❁ Kale	❁ Dandelion
❁ Spinach	Greens
❁ Arugula	❁ Broccoli
❁ Collard greens	❁ Brussel Sprouts
❁ Mixed Greens	❁ Cauliflower
❁ Frise Salad	❁ Cabbage
❁ Beet Greens	❁ Swiss Chard

Veggies and Starches

❈ Carrots	❈ Bell Peppers
❈ Parsnips	❈ Leeks
❈ Celery Root	❈ Zucchini
❈ Sweet Potato	❈ Eggplant
❈ Butternut Squash	❈ Artichokes
❈ Acorn Squash	❈ Asparagus
❈ Jicama	❈ Celery
❈ Onions	❈ Tomatoes
❈ Garlic	❈ Radicchio

Protein / Anti-inflammatory Spices & Herbs

Protein	Anti-inflammatory Spices & Herbs
❈ Legumes (beans, peas, lentils, chickpeas)	❈ Ginger root/powder
❈ Tofu	❈ Turmeric root/powder
❈ Tempeh	❈ Cinnamon
❈ Wild Fish	❈ Nutmeg
❈ Organic Meats	❈ Sage
❈ Nuts	❈ Cilantro
❈ Vegan Protein	❈ Basil
	❈ Parsley
	❈ Mint

Grains	Good Fats
❈ Quinoa ❈ Brown Rice ❈ Oats ❈ Wild Rice	❈ Olive Oil ❈ Avocado Oil ❈ Avocados ❈ Nuts butter ❈ Grass-fed butter ❈ Grapeseed Oil

Seeds	Sweets/ Sweetners
❈ Chia Seeds ❈ Hemps Seeds ❈ Hemp Seeds ❈ Goji berries ❈ Flax seeds ❈ Pine nuts ❈ Sunflower seeds ❈ Pumpkin seeds	❈ All kinds of fruits ❈ Raw Honey ❈ Agave Nectar ❈ Coconut Sugar/ Syrup ❈ Rice Syrup ❈ Pure Maple Syrup

Snacks	
❈ Hummus with tortilla chips or veggies ❈ Baby Carrots ❈ Celery Sticks ❈ Seaweed ❈ Rice Crackers ❈ Berries	❈ Banana ❈ Any fruits ❈ Apples w/nut butters ❈ Popcorn ❈ Goji Berries ❈ Figs

To make things easier for you, I have created a Healthy Zesty Meal Planning Template you can use for making your planning easier. Go to my website to download your free copy.

Download your FREE copy here:

http://healthyzesty.com/meal-planning-template

HEAL YOUR GUT - ACTION STEP 7

Supplement with Gut-Healing Natural Supplements

For more serious gut imbalances, where a damage of the gut lining might have occurred, integrative doctors and naturopaths recommend a more thorough approach, in which case introducing supplements known to promote healing of the gut lining might be needed.

L-glutamine and quercetin are known to be beneficial in such situations, but I recommend talking to an integrative doctor or a naturopath before starting such a supplement regimen.

But the changes you've made by now to your diet (by implementing the actionable tips discussed so far) are already having a positive impact on healing your gut, with or without these supplements. The supplements are just meant to aid in the healing process and speed up the repair of the gut lining in people with gut impermeability, known as leaky gut syndrome. This is something I personally used to supplement with during my recovery, on top of my changes in diet. If you are one of those people with more sensitive digestive systems and suspect gut damage, I suggest you talk to your doctor and get support throughout the healing process.

Go to www.healthyzesty.com/3-day-healthy-zesty-jumpstart-menu to download your 3-day menu!

HEAL YOUR GUT - ACTION STEP 8

Replay

To recap, the very first undertaking for healing your gut consisted of the elimination stage. The purpose of this stage was to remove common inflammatory foods from your diet and give your digestive system a break and even a chance to identify potential hidden food sensitivities that could have hindered your energy and mood without you even knowing it. While this is a temporary elimination (for at least two weeks), I recommend you go through such an elimination routine at least once a year in order to keep your body from overloading with food irritants, allergens, and toxins. Think of it as a cleanse, a detox for revitalizing your digestive system for better digestion and nutrients assimilation. At the end of the day, your gut will impact your energy and mood, so it is vital that you keep your gut happy and functioning at its best.

By implementing the tips outlined in this first part of the book for improving your Gut health, you are well on your way to feeling healthy and zesty. The actionable tips outlined so far should have taught you how to eat healthy, whole and clean, which is what keeps your Gut balanced and what a healthy-zesty diet is all about.

The truth is I could talk about Gut health and ways of healing your Gut for days, as I am living proof of the devastating effects an unbalanced Gut could have on your overall health. That's why healing the Gut is my main focus when coaching clients for improving their health, weight, and mood.

My hope is that the changes you made so far helped you understand the importance of healing your Gut, listening to your gut and what to feed your body for increased energy and wellbeing that lasts. Although this represents the principal part in achieving your ultimate goal of feeling healthy and zesty, this is not all. There is more that needs to come into balance for you to feel healthy and zesty and truly become the best version of yourself.

What follows is what feeds us at a deeper level, what we need to feel whole. I invite you to keep reading to discover the next steps for regaining your energy and living the life of your dreams.

Nurture Your Whole Self

It's true that food has a tremendous impact on how we feel and look. You know the saying "garbage in, garbage out". Therefore, eating clean, nutritious and whole foods is the first step in feeling and looking your best. But your journey to achieving that shouldn't stop there. I'd say it's equally important how you nurture your whole self. How you make room for inner joy, self-care and anything else that makes you feel complete.

Have you notice that when you feel happy, stress-free and playful your cravings are under control and you might not even feel hunger? Even if you eat less of a perfectly healthy meal and might even splurge a little bit on not so healthy occasional snacks, when you feel happy, connected and fulfilled the impact of the "not so perfect diet" is not as meaningful. Why? Because your body is fueled on a different, much deeper level. That's not to say that just because you feel happy you should splurge on eating junk. Your feelings of happiness and wellbeing will soon wear off, as you eat more and more junk. It won't take long until you start feeling that things that once used to make you feel good or happy will not have the same effect on you. That's because your energy will be depleted due to lack of proper nutrients and growing inflammation in your body, which will ultimately affect your mood, energy, and health.

The secret sits in achieving balance. Balance between eating healthy and nurturing your body, mind, and spirit. Which is why I personally promote healthy eating and balanced living! It's not one or the other. It's both. And while we all know what healthy eating looks like, balanced living could be different for each of us. But the common ground to balanced living for everyone is the practice of self-care. It is ultimately what we all crave and need in order to compensate for what we are lacking. It is a way of nurturing your whole self.

Self-care can come in the form of listening to our body and allowing ourselves time to rest, getting a massage, reading a book, walking, spending more time with the loved ones or even alone, watching a movie, meditating, meeting up with a friend, saying no to things that don't make us happy, or taking a long relaxing bath. These are just some examples of little things we should all do in order to take good care of ourselves inside and out and live a more fulfilled life. It is about putting ourselves first, as selfish as that sounds. At the end of the day, if we don't feel happy and vibrant our families won't either and they will suffer the consequences.

Now, on the other hand, think of a time when you felt crappy, and on top of that you poisoned your body with junk food to compensate for it. Instead of feeling better you felt even worse. You didn't give your body what it needed at the time, which could have been some form of self-care that could have filled the void, without the need to intoxicate your body.

Think of the times you were a child, playing outside with your friends the entire day without realizing you were hungry. You were happy playing and being surrounded by friends, feeling accepted as you were and not worrying about your future. That innocent state, without expectations and judgments, is our ideal state of being. The one that brings inner joy, peace, and the feeling of being connected to something bigger. While I know we can't relive our childhood, I think it is our right to feel happy, spoiled and loved, like we felt when we were kids. For that, I recommend that you think of yourself as a kid eager to be spoiled. Only this time it will be you spoiling yourself by attending to your own needs and taking time for yourself. Make this a daily, weekly or monthly ritual, whatever you can fit into your schedule. But do make a date with yourself and ask yourself what is that you need or crave and find a way to satisfy that. It doesn't have to be anything major. It could be something as easy as spending a long morning in bed without fixing breakfast for anyone, or savoring a glass of red wine while watching a romantic comedy, or breathing deeply.

At first sight, practicing self-care might seem a luxury and you might even think you don't have time for it. But trust me, you do! Time is, in essence, the only equalizer. We all have the same amount of time in a day. It's just a matter of better organizing your time, setting priorities and learning to say *No*. Once you become familiar with your needs and honor them, your energy will take off and new possibilities will unfold. Without realizing you will end up managing your time more efficiently because you will feel more satisfied, more energetic and happy. I dare you to try it for a week and notice the changes in how you feel and act.

After all, self-care is the foundation of living a satisfying and balanced life!

Healthy-Zesty Self-Care Tips

Consider implementing some or the following self-care tips to nourish your mind, body and spirit:

*Schedule 30 minutes alone time with yourself
(daily or every other day)*

We all need some alone time to decompress and connect with our inner thoughts and feelings.

If you are like me, you probably spend your day running around to take care of your family, do a good job at work, run errands, fix dinner (that's if you had time to plan for it), and commuting, all robbing us of precious time. You find yourself exhausted at the end of the day, wondering where your day went and if this is all there is to life – running like a robot, without any tangible reward.

I remember my doctor used to ask me, "What do you do for yourself? How do you spend 'me time'?" That question always left me speechless. Only when I was asked that question did I realize there was no such thing as "me time" left for me. "Who has time for such things?" I'd think to myself.

It took me years to understand the importance of this question and what was behind it. This was one of the drops that kept adding to the bucket of my own misery. It wasn't until I got really sick and later on focused on holistic healing that I changed my way of living and caring for myself at a deeper level. I realized there was more to self-care than just taking a shower, applying make-up and dressing up. There is so much more we can do for ourselves at a deeper level and it is my goal to help you make those changes in your own life and start taking yourself seriously. Your happiness and that of those around you depend on that!

You can spend this alone time any way you want. Whatever speaks to you that day - reading, reflecting over your day, making note of what went good and what not so good, writing in your journal, daydreaming, planning your next day or even planning dinner for the next 2 days.

Keep a Gratitude Journal

The power of gratitude is truly underestimated! Trust me, the more grateful you are for what you already have, the more things to be grateful for will come into your life. It's that simple!

Gratitude helps you focus on positive events, on what's good in your life and it raises your spirits and vibrations instantly.

Start by writing down at least 5 things you are grateful for each evening before you go to sleep. It could be any little thing such as being grateful for finding a parking spot closer to the building entrance (although I'd recommend parking farther away, as walking is good for you). You will see that over time your daily list will grow bigger and you will find more and more things to be thankful for while feeling lighter and happier.

So, what are you grateful for? Take a few minutes to think over your day and write down 5 good things that happened to you today. If you have a hard time identifying something good, just start by being grateful for your eyes that allow you to see your dear ones; for your hands that allow you to touch and hug your loved ones; for your legs that allow you to run or walk on this Earth; for your nose that allows you to smell the flowers; for being alive!

Daily Body Scrub

Body scrubbing could be done in the shower, or isolated from the shower, with a special scrubbing loofah, scrubbing gloves or just a hot towel.

As basic as this may sound, the process of scrubbing your body has a powerful physical, mental and emotional effect when done with intent and creates a deeper connection with yourself.

Benefits of Body Scrubbing [20]

- ❁ Improves your body circulation
- ❁ Promotes toxins elimination through the open pores
- ❁ Improves the appearance of your skin
- ❁ Calms your mind

20 © 2003 Integrative Nutrition Inc. (used with permission)

❋ Helps you become more intimate with your own self by discovering your ticklish points, your likes, and dislikes and learn to love your body.

❋ Boosts your overall mood and energy.

❋ Reduces muscle tension

❋ Re-energizes when done in the morning

❋ Deeply relaxes when done at night

❋ Softens deposits of hard fat below the skin and prepares them for discharge

❋ Allows excess fat, mucus, cellulite, and toxins to actively discharge to the surface rather than to accumulate around deeper vital organs

❋ Relieves stress through meditative action of rubbing the skin

❋ Activates the lymphatic system, especially when scrubbing underarms and groin

❋ Easy massage and deep self-care

❋ Can be a sacred moment in your day, especially if done with candlelight and a drop or two of essential oil such as lavender

❋ Creates a profound and loving relationship with the body, especially parts not often shown care, and particularly for a person with body image problems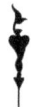

❋ Spreads energy through the chakras

If you choose to try the hot towel scrub, which is a process outside your regular shower, follow the directions below. This is something I learned at IIN and I find it a very calming ritual (but doing just the body scrubbing in the shower with a loofah or scrubbing gloves will be as satisfying, especially when in a hurry).

Directions for Performing the Hot Towel Scrub: [21]

- ❁ Turn on the hot water and fill the sink
- ❁ Hold the towel at both ends and place in the hot water
- ❁ Wring out the towel
- ❁ While the towel is still hot and steamy, begin to scrub the skin gently

- ❁ Scrub one section of the body at a time. For example, begin with the hands and fingers and work your way up the arms to the shoulders, neck, and face, then down to the chest, upper back, abdomen, lower back, buttocks, legs, feet, and toes

- ❁ Scrub until the skin becomes slightly pink or until each part becomes warm

- ❁ Reheat the towel often by dipping it in the sink of hot water after scrubbing each section or as soon as the towel starts to cool.

21 © 2003 Integrative Nutrition Inc. (used with permission)

Be Bad

Do you always play by the rules and like to please others? How about throwing away the rules and being "bad" for once? There is a certain feeling of joy and freedom that comes with letting your guard down every once in a while, and being "bad".

Pick a day a month, or a week, when you decide to be bad! And I don't mean hitting someone or committing a crime. I mean giving yourself a break, not being so hard on yourself and intentionally giving in to temptation or acting daring and childishly. Whatever could put a smile on your face and bring a sense of relief. Think of "bad" as something you think you shouldn't do or is irresponsible, but not compromising. It could be finally having that slice of chocolate cake you have been craving without judging your decision, buying yourself a gift, going one day without washing dishes, saying no to your boss, leaving work early and getting a massage, having a girl's night out. You decide what it will be. The idea is to do something that makes you feel free, happy and in control.

You will feel liberated and judgment free! It is a way of spicing up your life in a safe way, thus avoiding the risk of falling victim to dangerous cravings that could set in when your life is boring, restrictive, stressful or out of balance. We all need to find a way to decompress, laugh at our mistakes and just live a little. Otherwise, at some point, something in us will burst and bring with it unwanted consequences.

I have to confess you something – until recently, I'd never had a girls' night out (not after I got married, at least). I always refused any invitations I got from my colleagues at work, as I considered that to be an inappropriate behavior for someone married with children. Until one day after work when my female boss and also friend told me it was a work assignment for me to go out for drinks together. Since she was my boss, I thought I should obey, so I did. I remember even now the guilty feeling I had when I called home to announce I was going to be running late. But spending that evening outside my home with a friend, sharing girls stories over a glass of red wine and laughing at the silly guys working hard to get our attention, was exhilarating. That adrenaline rushing through my body was something I haven't experienced ever since I started dating. It completely pumped me up and kept me giggling for hours after I got home at the thought of doing something unusual, something that made me feel free and connected with my inner child. That's what we should all be reaching for and that's what made me realize how important it is we find ways to spice up our life with little "bad" things.

This type of approach is what I promote when it comes to eating healthy as well. I don't believe in a "one diet fits all," which is why I consider we should all be flexible in our approach to food and lifestyle to some degree. Otherwise, we could quickly fall off track and switch from extremely healthy eating to binge eating and uncontrollable cravings.

Same goes for lifestyle choices and self-care, which is why I think we should all be deliberately bad at times!

So, what are you waiting for? Go ahead and do something "bad" today! What will that be? Write it down in your journal and go do it!

Get a Massage

Human beings thrive on touch. We can't properly develop physically and emotionally without being held, caressed, kissed and touched. Think of a newborn baby. They cry for their mother's touch as soon as they come out of the womb. They need that so they feel safe.

As adults we are the same way, although we react differently to the lack of touch. We become insecure, resentful, depressed, isolated and may even develop serious health problems as a result. We crave being touched, but most of us don't know how to express that. Instead, we isolate ourselves, we immerse ourselves in our work, and we become unhappy and seek relief in food, alcohol or even worse, in drugs.

In order to satisfy this need of being touched, we should plan activities that involve touching. Lovemaking is one of such activities. But I know that's not always an option. Therefore, I highly recommend getting a professional massage once a month if possible or ask your partner to perform one for you once a week. Chances are, that may lead to something more that will satisfy your need of touch and connection on different levels as well. This is a win-win solution!

STEP THREE

Eliminate Toxic Relationships

"What do relationships have to do with how I feel and look?" you must think. Well, everything.

Our relationships shape who we are today, how we live our life, how we react to certain events, how we feel about ourselves and ultimately how happy we are.

If we live in a toxic relationship that makes us unhappy, we won't feel healthy no matter how healthy our diet is and how much kale we eat. Our relationships go through our Gut and impact our overall wellbeing as well.

When I say relationships I don't refer to your partner exclusively. I really mean anything that makes up your social circle, your social life: family, community, co-workers, friends and significant other.

Try to stay away from negative people and surround yourself with supporting people – people who share the same beliefs, who you have common interests with and lift up your spirits.

Have you ever noticed how you feel after a conversation with a negative person, who always complains, who always has a problem for every solution? Do you feel drained, sluggish and maybe even depressed? This is the effect of the negative energy that person lays on you, which brings down your vibrations.

Instead, when you run into a genuinely optimistic person, even if you only spoke for a couple of minutes, you already feel pumped with energy. Your vibrations were raised by that encounter and you are more optimistic and happy yourself.

We, humans, are social beings and we need to interact with others, so we feel connected. We need to feel part of a group, a community that cares for our wellbeing. That could be our family, church, school, workplace, or any other specialty groups for like-minded people. We feel happier and more connected and fulfilled when we have someone to share our accomplishments or sorrows with.

Think of it this way - what is the point to reach certain accomplishments and milestones in life if you have no one to share your success with? No one you can show off to?

I always like to share this joke with my friends and clients when I touch on this subject. It is a joke I heard when I was a teenager, but it didn't really hit home until later in life when my husband and I moved to the States and found ourselves without any family or close friends. No one we could brag or complain to without judgment.

So here goes the joke:

Following a major shipwreck, a young man ended up on a deserted island. He was all by himself not knowing what to do when all of a sudden a beautiful young lady appeared out of nowhere. The young lady was a well-known international model at the time, Claudia Shiffer, a beauty idol for most man. The young man was the happiest he could be to share the island with Claudia Shiffer alone and they eventually started an intimate relationship. A couple of days later the young man started feeling sad and not even Claudia Shiffer's presence would make him happy. Claudia Shiffer confused, asked him what was the matter. The young man then answered, "What is the point in having sex with Claudia Shiffer, the most beautiful woman in the world, if I can't brag about it to anyone?"

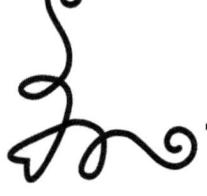
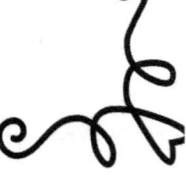

Joke aside, the truth is that we are all social beings in need of social interaction and deeper connection.

We have an innate need of feeling connected, accepted, needed and loved. Satisfying this hunger for healthy relationships and an active social life feeds us on a deeper emotional level than food. By satisfying this *Primary Food*[22], our need for actual food becomes secondary. As a result, when we feel happy and fulfilled at a personal level (thanks to practicing self-care and nurturing healthy relationships) we eliminate the need for junk food and even junky relationships. On the contrary, when this is something that's missing from our life we tend to fill that void by over-eating.

The Result?

A vicious circle starts. We gain weight, we lose our energy, we are unhappy and later on depressed.

Although we live in a world dominated by social media, our society today is deficient in social interaction. The more we rely on Facebook and other social media to satisfy our need of socializing the farther we get from actual socialization, which is vital to our sense of well-being and connection.

In my opinion, Facebook tends to put more pressure on us by making us compare ourselves and our lives with what others share on Facebook. We are encouraged to use Facebook as a tool to show off – look

22 ©2005 Integrative Nutrition Inc. (used with permission)

what I'm eating today; look where I am; look at my new dress. And on the other end of Facebook, there will be a few of us thinking how fortunate those people are and how miserable we are. It's so easy to deceive your friends on Facebook by posting a picture that depicts a perfect life, perfect relationships or a perfect body. But how about showing the real you? Accepting that life is not perfect and we all have our ups and downs? Who do you share that with? Do you dare to post that on Facebook, knowing it doesn't depict a perfect life or compete to that of others?

I don't know about you, but nowadays, thanks to Facebook, my friends don't even bother to pick up the phone to wish me happy birthday on my birthday. It's so much more convenient for them to just send a quick happy birthday in writing on Facebook. While I am appreciative of the fact they did acknowledge my special day, I must say it's not as impactful as a face to face encounter or phone call. That day used to be the day when I would get to talk to most of my old friends and family and share the latest events in my life, good and bad. I used to feel special and connected, even if for just one short day.

I want to believe we all feel the same way to some degree. I know we all might have a few of those "friends" we are happy to avoid talking to, some days, and that's when Facebook comes in handy. But we should not rely solely on Facebook for the most part of our social life. We need to connect on a deeper level, move away from the cyber social life and start living. You don't need to have hundreds of friends, like you have on Facebook, to have a fulfilled social life. A hand full of true friends and like-minded people is all you need to feel accepted, connected and cared for. But that doesn't mean you should toss away your Facebook account. That has its pros as well. However, it should not replace your real social life, but just add to it and spice it up a bit.

Tips for Cultivating Healthy Relationships

Spend time with supportive and positive people.

They lift your spirits up and help you see the half-full part of the glass. When you spend time with positive people you feel energized and ready to conquer the world.

Minimize the time spent with negative, draining people.

They spoil your mood and pull you down too. Make a conscious decision to step away from negative conversations. Excuse yourself or just smoothly change the subject. It's better to be alone than in bad company.

Spend alone time with your partner (if married or engaged).

Plan an outing with your partner alone at least once a month. Make it something special. Even if at first you might feel like you don't have a lot to talk about, other than just your kids, rest assured that you will soon rediscover the connection you once had before the kids were in the picture. In some way, it is like learning about each other once again. This will put a spark on your relationship and strengthen the bond.

Plan double dates.

It is still amazing to me what a positive impact a double date has on a couple. It's like an infusion of romantic energy, friendly competition, and seduction. You are forced to show the best part of you to your partner since you are now closely observed by the other couple as well, and if nothing else, you want to showcase your loving relationship. More often than not, this kind of outings lead to being more intimate with each other and add the spark back into the bedroom.

Plan social activities at least once a month.

This is more of a general outing, to various events where all eyes are not necessarily on you, but you get to mingle and meet new people.

Play games with your partner, family, and friends often.

It keeps you feeling young and brings out the child in you. You will feel happy, playful and reenergized in an instance. Plus, competition provides a boost of adrenaline that adds to your state of euphoria. Schedule a game night with your family or friends. Take turns in organizing game nights at each other's place, say, once a month.

Girls night out/boys night out is a must.

We need to spend time with friends and laugh with each other or even cry on each other's shoulder when need be.

Find your tribe.

Join a group of like-minded individuals (depending on your passions, interests, and field of work). When you are surrounded by like-minded people you feel understood, connected and supported in ways no others could. Sometimes, it's hard to feel entirely supported by your family, your coworkers or even your significant other, and that's when finding your tribe comes in handy.

Get in touch with your childhood friends.

Friendships made in childhood are probably the most sincere ones. It's amazing how easy it is to rekindle an old friendship made in childhood and feel completely safe and connected with that person even after 10 years apart. You feel as if you can talk about anything and everything without feeling judged. Those childhood friends know the real essence of you, the person you truly are, without adulthood concealers. They might be the best ones to listen to you and give you meaningful advice when in trouble.

Foster an open communication policy.

Communicate with your family and close friends often, whether in person or over the phone. Address issues as they arise and don't wait for them to build up, as they affect your health.

Don't hold grudges with anyone.

Learn to forgive others and yourself, so you can heal on the inside. If you don't have the courage to talk about it with the person you want to forgive, then write a letter and you decide if you want to send it or not. Just let it out and make more room for positive emotions in your heart.

View everyone you meet with gratitude.

They will sense your good intentions and they will be drawn to you, to your good vibe.

Focus on what's good in your life.

This way you attract more of the good stuff into your life and push away negativity.

Limit time on Facebook and other social media.

This might keep you away from spending quality face-to-face time with your dear ones.

Set an electronics-free day.

Proclaim an electronics-free day a month and stick to it. This goes for the entire household. However, be prepared for pushbacks from your kids, especially if you have teenagers (even if they are typically quiet, you will really hear their voices now!). Looking on the bright side, though, by going electronics-free you will be forced to be more present and connected with those around you and you'll end up spending quality time with your family. At the end of the day, even your kids will thank you and you might even hear them say: "this was fun!"

Say "I love you", "thank you" and "sorry" often!

These simple phrases do wonders in your relationship with others and yourself. Use these phrases when communicating with your family multiple times a day (especially "I love you") and learn to love and forgive yourself as well.

Experiment with these tips and notice what works best for you. What do you sense puts you in the best mood and boosts your connection with others? Repeat this often and plan in advance. But there should always be room for spontaneity too!

Remember that healthy relationships are not limited to your love life or family. It's about community and finding your tribe. Feeling part of a community and having a group of good friends are both key to a good health and happy life.

Go to www.healthyzesty.com/3-day-healthy-zesty-jumpstart-menu to download your 3-day menu!

STEP FOUR

Love Your Work

I never realized how much of an impact our work could have on our overall health and well-being until I got really sick and later on decided to take a break and changed my career.

Like most people used to say, I thought that a job was just that - a job. So why would that matter that much? We just go to work to get a paycheck and live the life we want, right? Well, not quite.

We spend the majority of our life at work, not with our families or living the life we want, unless our work really makes up the life we want, in which case we are some happy campers. And since we spend the biggest chunk of our time at work, we need to **find work we love, or learn to love the work we do!** [23] This is something I learned later in my healing process, thanks to my teacher at the Institute for Integrative Nutrition®, Joshua Rosenthal.

What I really think makes a big difference in our level of satisfaction with our job is aligning our work with our own beliefs and personality. When our career is in line with who we truly are, our job becomes a

---

23 (Rosenthal)

natural manifestation of our true essence. That's when we are in sync with our spiritual being and start living from our creative core, which opens up the space for new possibilities.

A recent study published in the Business News Daily shows that work affects our health on different levels. [24] It's not only the fact that we might be doing a job we don't like, or that doesn't fulfill us, that makes us sick, but also certain behaviors related to our work, such as:

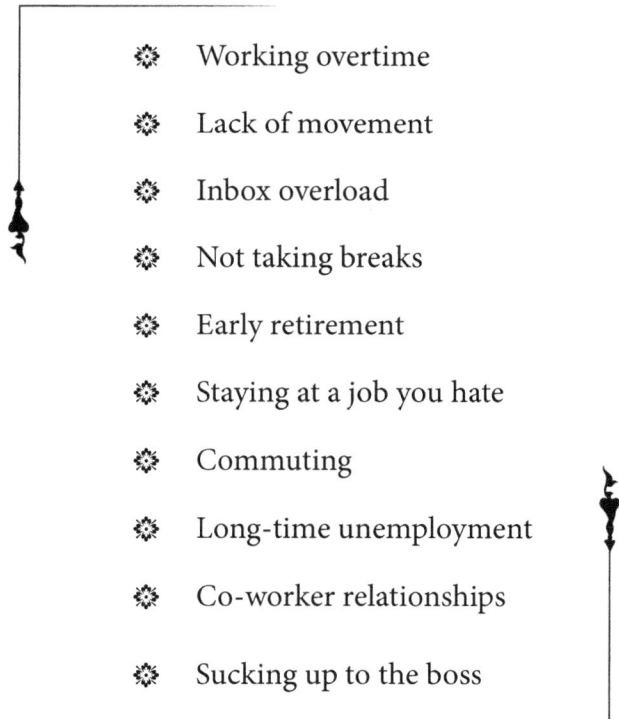

- ❈ Working overtime
- ❈ Lack of movement
- ❈ Inbox overload
- ❈ Not taking breaks
- ❈ Early retirement
- ❈ Staying at a job you hate
- ❈ Commuting
- ❈ Long-time unemployment
- ❈ Co-worker relationships
- ❈ Sucking up to the boss

You can read the entire details of the study here: http://www.business-newsdaily.com/2382-job-health-impact.html.

You can probably already identify yourself with at least a few of these behaviors, whether you thought about them this way or not. But the reality is, we need to be more mindful of our work behaviors and the effect work has on our life and therefore health. We live in a society where everything revolves around our work. Therefore, we live to work and not the other way around. Something has got to change!

As I mentioned in the beginning of this book, up until 4 years ago when I got seriously ill, I thought my career was the most important thing – after my family, of course. My struggle at the time was not having the energy to spend quality time with my little one after work. Despite my lack of energy and that persistent feeling of something missing from my life, I kept going, running after something that was not really what I wanted deep down, or who I truly was.

Because of my upbringing and the culture I was raised in, I never thought I had the right to complain or that a job should be more than just a job. So, instead of chasing a dream, I was chasing a promotion, hoping that will bring me closer to my dream. Only to realize, that with each promotion I would get more stressed, more unhappy and less time for myself and my family. There was no balance anymore. So I started wondering what was the point? What was I really chasing? What was the final destination and was it really worth it? I then realized that my biggest problem was not loving the work I was doing, the environment I was in, the way I was affecting other people's life as a result of my actions. Because I was successful at what I was doing I thought I had to carry on, but never allowed myself to attach any feelings to my work, like I didn't have the right to even question myself about such a thing. I was actually afraid to even mention my discontent with my job to my family and friends. I remember my sister commenting after I left my job, "But I thought you loved your job? You were doing so well and never thought you were not happy." And that's because I never allowed my feelings to control me. And that's another problem when it comes to your health – concealing your feelings and letting them eat you out from within.

I remember how I ran into a friend about a year after I changed careers and started dedicating myself to health and wellness coaching. He made a sweet comment about how I was looking so much better and younger. My answer was simple – "It must be because for once in my life I am doing something I love doing, something that fulfills me at a deeper level"

For me, the biggest problem was not feeling I was helping anyone, not making a difference. I felt I was put on this Earth for a purpose, but I just didn't know what that was yet. I needed a wake-up call for this realization to happen. I figured, since I was so lucky to discover the cancer early in the process and heal completely, there must be a reason this had happened. I am a firm believer that everything happens for a reason.

As for my enlightenment, I must say it didn't happen overnight. It was a process that started taking shape as soon as I began questioning myself and gradually worked toward developing my self-awareness. Only then you can reach that point of discovering your inner self, your true nature, your deepest desires, and purpose.

So I invite you to reflect on where you are now and where you would like to be. How does your work make you feel, knowing it has a direct effect on your long term health?

Do you love the work you do? If so, identify what is that you love about it and try to make room for more of that into your work life.

If you don't love the work you do, what can you do to make it more appealing? What can you change? What would you like to be different? How can you put those changes into action?

Just take some time to write down the answers to these questions and reflect on them. The goal for this exercise is not that you quit your job. Not by any means. This exercise will help you get some insight into your life, your likes, and dislikes and will help you identify some action steps that could get you closer to your desired life.

Tips for Getting Clarity on Your Ideal Work

If you are still uncertain about what you like to do, what makes you happy and fulfilled career-wise, try to answer the following questions. Write your answers in the space below or in a journal.

What makes me laugh?

_____

_____

_____

_____

What is my biggest strength?

_____

_____

_____

_____

What is my main weakness?

_____

_____

_____

_____

What did I use to play as a child?

_____

_____

_____

_____

What type of activity makes time stop when I immerse myself in?

_____

_____

_____

What kind of people do I like to be surrounded by?

_____

_____

_____

_____

What do most people say I do well?

_____

_____

_____

_____

Identify a few words or phrases that describe your personality?

_____

_____

_____

_____

How do I like to be seen by others?

_____

_____

_____

_____

If I could do anything without worrying about money, what would that be?

_____

_____

_____

_____

After you answered all these questions, reflect on your answers and brainstorm on potential job options that would fit these characteristics, or identify ways in which you can utilize these traits in your current job. This will add to your personal satisfaction and sense of accomplishment for doing what you love so that it doesn't feel as much like a job anymore. Make it fun and rewarding.

Just remember, when what you do matches your personality and is in sync with your true self, everything falls into place and your job doesn't feel like a job, but an extension of who you truly are. That's when magic happens!

Tips for Making a Career Change and Finding Work You Love

If this exercise helped you define what it is that you would like to do and you've determined you need a change, here are some tips I learned at IIN ® that helped me follow through with my career change: [25]

❁ Research the career options you narrowed down and determine if there are any additional qualifications you might need.

❁ If your ideal job is withing the same company, but different field, start talking to various leaders in the company who could help on a project and showcase your work ethic and enthusiam this way. This is more powerful to a hiring manager than an impressive resume. I personally welcomed this approach when in a hiring manager role.

❁ Join professional organizations related to your desired career. Attend social events and start networking.

❁ Reach out to people working in your desired field and ask for their guidance and support. Most people like to talk about themselves and share their stories.

25 (Rosenthal)

❧ Reach out to prospective employers and make your intentions heard. Be professional, courteous and show your enthusiasm. Even if they don't have an opening, they could still add you to their list and be among the first to know when a new opportunity comes along.

❧ Don't give up your job until you have a back-up plan (unless you have serious reasons to do so). Being jobless could add more stress and affect your health even more if money becomes a problem.

❧ Be patient. Changing careers or finding a new job takes time. Just keep an open mind and visualize your ideal job and happy life often. This will help you stay positive and not lose hope. Trust that something good is about to happen, and it will!

Don't forget, "It's all about finding work you love, or learning to love the work you do." (Joshua Rosenthal) [26]

---

26 (Rosenthal)

STEP FIVE

Move Your Body

Moving your body is a must for a healthy mind, body, and spirit. But do you really take this to heart?

Time and time again, science has proven the health benefits of an active lifestyle. It's really not a myth.

Benefits of Exercising [27]

- ✿ Aids in digestion

- ✿ Promotes regular elimination (colon health)

- ✿ Improves circulation

- ✿ Reduces inflammation

- ✿ Boosts metabolism and promotes weight loss

- ✿ Supports a healthy heart

- ✿ Boosts stamina

---

27 © Integrative Nutrition Inc.(used with permission)

- Triggers the feel good hormones (there is nothing like the runner's high)

- Fights anxiety

- Promotes healthy respiratory system

- Improves sex drive

- Improves immune function

- Promotes healthy, glowing skin

- Improves focus

- Lowers the chances of developing osteoporosis

- Enhances quality of sleep

- Improves mood and overall sense of well-being

Lots of reasons to take exercising seriously!

When it comes to leading a healthy lifestyle, most of us think of eating healthy but forget that moving our body is also part of a healthy lifestyle. Exercising should not be seen as a chore, as a seasonal or occasional activity, but should become part of our lifestyle. The secret, though, is to not look at it as just that – exercising. The idea is to move your body often and find a way of doing so that matches your lifestyle.

Most of us have probably tried multiple forms of exercising but couldn't stick to them long term because they didn't fit our lifestyle or didn't come naturally.

What I always tell my clients in my health coaching sessions, when discussing the importance of moving their body, is that they should always try to build a new exercise routine upon an already existing and well-established habit. This way this new exercise routine is easier to stick to without second guessing our will and becomes an ingrained habit in no time.

For instance, up until 2 years ago, my main exercise routine was limited to occasional yoga. Although I was attempting to go to the yoga studio twice a week, I rarely managed to actually do yoga more than just once a week, because of the time of the day I'd chosen to engage in such activities.

However, when a move to Germany for a year changed my schedule, everything else changed too. Once in Germany, I found it very difficult to find a yoga studio where they would actually teach in English, so yoga was not an option for me anymore. I was now living in the city, where I was walking everywhere, so this was a plus, but I didn't want to stop there. I felt I needed something more, so I started running. At first, I could not run for more than just 10 minutes, but I kept building up my endurance every day until I managed to run for 30 minutes without stopping.

The secret?

I chose to attach this activity to something that was already ingrained in my daily routine. Every morning I had to walk my daughter to the school bus. So every morning when I woke up I put my running outfit on without even thinking, fixed breakfast, packed lunch and headed out the door with my little one ready for my morning run, rain or shine. I'd kiss her goodbye and off I went.

I'd gone from no running to running for 30 minutes a day, five days a week, in less than a month. Once I got to this point where it became a routine, I felt I couldn't live without it. It was like a drug, like something was missing if I went for more than 2 days without running, without catching that breath of fresh air that got my adrenaline going and energy rushing through my body. I was now ready for a productive and positive day! My entire outlook on life, energy, mood, and focus improved when I kept my body moving, which is why the addiction that comes with it and the withdrawal symptoms we experience when not being active.

Tips for Moving Your Body

Identify an already existing daily routine that you can attach a new exercise routine to and stick to it.

Find an exercise activity you enjoy; something you can stick to for a while. Everybody is different and while running might be the best exercise for me, walking or biking might be more suitable for you. Experiment with different types of exercises. There is no wrong or right. You decide what works best for you. And don't be afraid to alternate routines, so you don't get bored easily.

Think of what you liked to do as a child in order to identify an enjoyable activity you are more likely to stick to.

Move your body at least 20 minutes a day, 5 days a week, or 30 minutes a day, 3 days a week. It could be just a simple brisk walk for 20 minutes. Walk like you are in a hurry, so that your heart rate reaches a healthy target rate. In order to calculate your target heart rate subtract your age from 220. That should be the maximum heart rate you should target to reach when performing an aerobic exercise.

Ditch the elevator. Take the stairs when you have an option.

Park your car as far away from the building entrance as possible when going to work or shopping. Any additional walking benefits your body.

Find a fitness pal. Some people are more motivated to stick to a routine when they are accompanied by a friend.

Move your body naturally. Find ways to move your body without following an exercise routine. Walk through the city, mall, in the neighborhood or in the park. Whenever you have some free time or feel stressed and tired choose to get out and take some fresh air. The more tired you feel the more you need to exercise, even if it seems hard to believe and even harder to do it. You will see that once you start moving your energy is stimulated and you start feeling better in an instance. And the best part is that your energy will be at its peak even hours after.

Remember that our ancestors didn't have to go to the gym to stay fit and active. What kept them fit, healthy and active was their lifestyle. On the other hand, our current lifestyle – dominated by automation and engineering of every activity that once required some level of physical effort – is what is forcing us to be less physically active. We now have to set aside special time for scheduled physical activities that are challenging to keep up with and thus we end up giving up before we managed to turn them into ingrained habits.

What's more, depending on where we live, our reliance on driving everywhere, instead of walking, adds to our waistline, our health issues and thus, misfortune. Ever wondered why people in Europe, such as France, eat bread, cheese, foie gras and drink wine, but still manage to keep a fit figure? They move their body regularly by walking almost everywhere. That by itself takes care of the need to schedule extra time daily for gym or other physical activities and leaves more time for enjoying it with family and friends. This, too, adds to an individual's sense of wellbeing. They have more time to laugh, go out and truly enjoy life. Having a rich and satisfying social life enriches our purpose and makes us feel happier and thus healthier. So, when you can, opt for moving your body naturally and free up time for the fun stuff. You owe that to yourself, to your desire for a healthy and zesty life!

Go to www.healthyzesty.com/3-day-healthy-zesty-jumpstart-menu to download your 3-day menu!

STEP SIX

Tap Into Your Life Purpose

The last step in the program that completes the path to a healthy-zesty life and makes us feel whole is finding our purpose; the reason for waking up in the morning and putting up with all that life throws at us, good and bad. When you have a purpose and live your life driven by it everything falls into place, effortlessly.

There is nothing worse than feeling you don't have a purpose. Lack of clarity around our purpose could make us feel sad, depressed, affect our health and digestion and even make us crave junk foods. Our body has to compensate somehow for what it lacks and more often than not it will mistake that lack of purpose and joy in our life with lack of food. And here we are again eating our sadness away and entering a vicious circle: emotional eating results in gaining weight, which in turns makes us sick, more depressed and we binge eat again hoping to make that feeling go away.

Lack of purpose is related to lack of clarity, which in turn relates back to our Gut. When our gut is out of balance it affects not only our digestion and our weight but our energy, our motivation, and moods, which is why the gut is now considered our second brain, as discussed in the first part of this book.

This last step brings us full circle to where we started, to the foundation of a healthy-zesty life: our Gut. Once we start caring for our Gut and eating real food, our Gut will function at its best and do what it's meant to: digest food, absorb nutrients, give us energy, protect us against diseases and mediate our mood and focus.

I know this sounds idealistic and not many people feel they live a purposeful life. That's either because they still don't know what their purpose is, or they know, but they didn't yet find a way to align their work or their life with their higher purpose. But what I know for sure is that finding your purpose, the reason to wake up in the morning, is what feeds your higher self; what gives you the drive for leading a healthier and happier life. Whether you find something to live for beyond your job or make your job and purpose work together it doesn't really matter that much. When you know your purpose, your actions are driven by it and your life becomes richer and more meaningful. That's when your career becomes secondary. Your focus shifts from your career to your purpose and great things start to happen. You are now in sync with your spiritual being and start living from your creative core, which opens up the space for new possibilities.

According to an article published in National Geographic, research revealed that having a sense of purpose increases the life expectancy by up to 7 years.[28] For me, this is yet another confirmation that having a purpose, something worth living for, directly impacts the quality of our life.

I remember envying those people who I thought found their higher purpose and managed to lead their life driven by that purpose and even make a living out of it. At that time, I felt purposeless and somewhat lost. I didn't have a clear target, a real definition of what success or happiness would mean to me. That's how it feels when you are not living from your core, when you are not connected with your higher self, with your higher purpose. And that's where I was up until 3 years ago.

My own story made me realize that we all need a sort of a wake-up call for us to change; for us to become more self-aware and grounded; for us to be present in the moment, but mindful of our future target. That's when we are in tune with our spiritual self and live from our core. Our actions are then driven by more than just habits or necessity, they are driven by our purpose, by what makes us happy and whole, by what makes us want to wake up in the morning and keep trying. And that, my friend, is what living life with purpose means. That's what contributes to living a healthy and zesty life!

You probably wonder now how you can find your purpose if you haven't found it already. I won't lie to you and tell you this is something that happens overnight. However, I can tell you how to flex the muscles of your own awareness, so you can get closer to finding or defining your purpose.

---

28 (National Geographic)

On the other hand, even if you now feel you haven't found your purpose, that's already inside of you. You just didn't take the time to process it and become aware of it or didn't say it out loud yet. And that's perfectly fine; it's not too late. Wherever you are now is enough and you are enough.

Your purpose doesn't have to be anything big like saving the world, but something that defines you and makes you happy. Something that motivates you to get over a boring task or a difficult event, knowing that there is a light at the end of the tunnel. It could be something as simple as feeling part of a community and being surrounded by friends. As long as that is something that resonates with you. Maybe you grew up in a large family, where you always had company and felt supported. You are now living in a different part of the world and still crave that connection. So you know that deep down you would like to have that type of community around you. Therefore, your purpose might be related to this desire of yours for being surrounded by people, feeling loved and accepted. You now know this is your purpose, what makes you tick and your actions will be led by this inner desire.

To me, finding or defining our purpose requires believing in something bigger than ourselves and developing self-awareness. Therefore, I recommend two ways in which you can get closer to defining your purpose:

- By tapping into your spirituality
- By developing self-awareness

Tapping into Your Spirituality

For centuries people found relief in putting their fate into something bigger, something out of their control that gave them hope; hope that someone or something was looking after them and pushing them forward.

Whether you believe that higher power exists or not, finding a practice that connects you with your higher self and brings you a sense of inner peace will make life more meaningful.

Studies show that people who join a faith-based community tend to live longer by 4 to 14 years than people who don't. [29]

I don't know whether it is the actual faith or the sense of belonging to a community that makes such a big impact, but I like to think it's a combination of the two. What I do know, though, is that when you have faith in something it's easier to get over your fears and find strength when dealing with difficult situations. This by itself contributes to boosting your optimism and staying positive, which in turn fuels your health and happiness. It must be the power of positive psychology!

When it comes to spirituality, there are 3 options that could fit the purpose. You don't have to be religious to be able to explore this side of you. You decide what truly speaks to you and brings you that sense of connection you need for feeling whole. Explore the 3 options below and decide on implementing one or all of them if you are not already doing so:

29 (National Geographic)

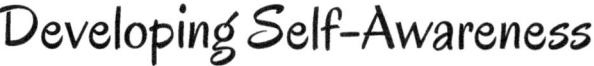

- ❊ Join a faith-based community or just choose to pray to a higher power you believe in.

- ❊ Practice meditation. This helps you develop self-awareness, connect with your higher self and get clear on your purpose.

- ❊ Spend alone time in nature and focus on the sense of endless space while connecting with your higher self.

Developing Self-Awareness

Like I said before, up until 3 years ago I didn't know what my purpose was. I was unhappy with my life. I felt tired all the time and I was living life like a robot without any clear goal or expectation. I was at a point where I wasn't in tune with my higher self and purpose and therefore, I felt unhappy and disconnected. It took a wakeup call for me to realize I was missing something. I was missing the purpose, the why that would make my life more exciting. I just didn't have the clarity and self-awareness needed to find my purpose. Acknowledging this was the first step I took for cultivating my self-awareness. Once I learned to pay attention to my internal signals, to what made me tick and filled me with joy and hope for the future, I became aware of my true purpose, my reason to wake up in the morning with excitement. So many people in this world suffer from chronic diseases that could easily be prevented with proper nutrition and self-care. By inspiring others and teaching them make better choices for a healthier life I know I am making a difference in reducing the epidemic of chronic disease and creating a ripple effect for a healthier, happier community!

I am telling you this story because I want to stress out that finding your purpose, doing what you love and living a healthy-zesty life starts and ends with self-awareness. And like I said before, self-awareness is not something you develop overnight, but something you cultivate over time with practice. It is my hope that the tips below will help you develop your sense of self and give you more insight into your own purpose, your "why".

How to Develop Self-Awareness and be More In Tune with Your Higher Self

Ask yourself these questions and write your answers below or in a journal:

What is that I love to do?

_____

_____

_____

_____

What makes me happy?

_____

_____

_____

_____

What type of activity makes time stay still when I dedicate myself to it?

_____

_____

_____

_____

What am I good at?

_____

_____

_____

_____

What others say often I am good at?

_____

_____

_____

_____

What is my biggest hobby? How could I make money from practicing my hobby?

_____

_____

_____

_____

If I could be anything what would I be?

_____

_____

_____

_____

If I knew the answer, what would that be?

_____

_____

_____

_____

These types of questions will help you get to know yourself a bit better. They will make you think out of the box and not just assume a status quo. They will lead you to the real you, the real purpose that could potentially bring balance in your life.

Practice Meditation

I can't say enough about the benefits of meditation. It is a practice that, if done frequently and consistently, has miraculous healing powers. Not only is meditation a promotor of self-awareness, but it is known to have many other health benefits. According to an article published by the Chopra Center, here are some of the benefits of meditation I want to share with you: [30]

Relief from stress and anxiety (meditation mitigates the effects of the fight-or-flight response, decreasing the production of stress hormones such as cortisol and adrenaline)

❈ Decreased blood pressure and hypertension

❈ Lower cholesterol levels

❈ More efficient oxygen use by the body

❈ Increased production of the anti-aging hormone DHEA

❈ Restful sleep

❈ Improved concentration and clarity

❈ Journaling

---

30 (Chopra Center)

Journaling

This is another way to get more in-tune with your higher-self and purpose. Write down the answers to the questions highlighted earlier in the section above. Write the first thing that comes to your mind without any filter. Let your mind run free without any judgment or fear. This is for your own eyes only. Aside, write anything else that troubles you or comes to mind. Do this as often as you need to, but at least once a week, so you keep the creating juices going and get in touch with your desires. It's going to be much easier to actually make them a reality if you know exactly what they are and you put them out into the Universe.

All of these practices have the benefit of releasing stress and promoting a healthier and happier life when coupled with healthy eating and balanced living. So I hope you start experimenting with these and watch your healthy-zesty life unfold!

Go to www.healthyzesty.com/3-day-healthy-zesty-jumpstart-menu to download your 3-day menu!

Part Three

Conclusion

CONCLUSION

Overview of the 6 Pillars

The 6 steps I've highlighted throughout this book are a result of the 6 pillars I identified as important for living a happy, healthy and well-rounded life. They are the foundation of my program for overcoming exhaustion and achieving vibrant health. Let's recap and summarize the essence of the 6 pillars.

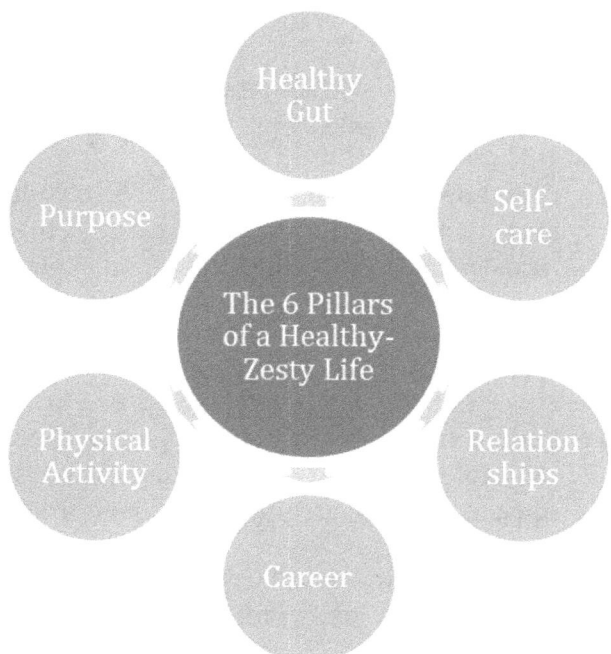

Gut Health

Your Gut is responsible for your overall wellbeing. A balanced Gut sets the foundation for a healthy digestion, which is the driver behind how we feel and even look. Your journey on the path to a healthy-zesty life starts here! This is the first and most important step for overcoming exhaustion and achieving vibrant health.

Key Points for Gut Health

- ❋ Reset digestion by eliminating food irritants and reducing toxic load.

- ❋ Balance intestinal flora with probiotic and pre-biotic rich foods and supplements.

- ❋ Maintain an 85/15 ratio of good vs. bad bacteria.

- ❋ Eat clean, whole foods and crowd out processed foods and refined sugars.

- ❋ Add more fresh fruits and vegetable to your diet for added fiber, iron, and antioxidants. This will leave less room for unhealthier food choices.

- ❋ Sugar is addicting, stripes away good flora and creates gut imbalances.

- ❋ Reduce sugar cravings by eating naturally sweet vegetables, such as sweet potatoes, butternut squash, carrots, parsnips, beets, celery root.

- ❋ Drink more water to flush out toxins and help your system detoxify more efficiently.

❀ Support digestion with bitters and digestive enzymes.

❀ Experiment with home cooked meals and reduce exposure to restaurant food, especially, fast foods.

❀ *Joshua's 90-10 Diet* - eat right most of the time, but allow yourself the liberty to be bad and indulge yourself at times without guilt.

❀ Supplement with gut healing supplements, such as L-glutamine and quercetin.

❀ Go through an elimination period at least once a year to revitalize your digestive system.

Self-Care

It's vitally important not only what you feed your body, but how you nurture your whole self.

The goal is to achieve a balance between eating healthy and nurturing your body, mind, and spirit, so you feel balanced and whole. If you don't take the time to nourish and love yourself nobody else will. When you love your body and let others see that you truly honor your whole self, those around you will respect and love you even more.

Key Points for Self-Care

❈ Schedule 30 minutes alone time with yourself (daily or every other day) in order to decompress and get more intimate with your needs and deepest desires.

❈ Practice gratitude. Gratitude helps you focus on positive events, on what's good in your life and it raises your spirits and vibrations instantly. When you are grateful for what you already have you create more space for getting more things to be grateful for.

❈ Stimulate body circulation by scrubbing your body daily. The process of scrubbing your body has a powerful physical, mental and emotional effect when done with intent and creates a deeper connection with yourself.

❈ Allow yourself to be "bad". There is a certain feeling of joy and freedom that comes with letting your guard down every once in a while, and being "bad". Every once in a while make a conscious decision to do something that feels a bit wild, or outside your typical boundaries (but don't get yourself in trouble).

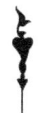

❁   Spoil yourself with a massage. As humans, we crave touch and being loved. Getting a massage is a perfect way of satisfying this need.

Relationships

As social beings, we base our lives on building relationships. The quality of our relationships impacts how we feel and how we react to certain events and circumstances. We process relationships through our gut as well. Therefore, no matter how much kale you eat, toxic relationships could still make you sick.

Key Points for Healthy Relationships

❁   Surround yourself with positive and supporting people. They lift you up and fuel you with energy in an instant.

❁   Avoid negative people, as they drag you down.

❁   Make time for time alone with your partner. Don't let that special connection you once had go down the drain.

❁   Practice and encourage communication with your family members, so you avoid turning a small misunderstanding into a bigger issue.

❋ Meet up with friends and family regularly to keep your need of socializing satisfied.

❋ Satisfy the child in you by engaging in playful activities. Plan game nights with friends or play sports games with your family in the backyard.

❋ Don't hold grudges with anyone. Learn to forgive others and yourself, so you can heal on the inside and make room for healthier relationships.

❋ Minimize time on social media and make room for more face to face time.

❋ Say "I love you", "thank you" and "sorry" often!

Career

Your job is where you spend most of your awake time, so it goes without saying that you need to love what you do, or find work you love. Your work, just like your relationships, impact the way you feel and could eventually make you sick if you hate it.

Key Points for a Satisfying Career

❋ Aim for aligning your work with your own beliefs and personality. When your career is in line with who you truly are, your job becomes a natural manifestation of your true essence.

❈ Practice journaling for deepening your self-awareness and discovering your calling.

❈ Network with people in fields that interest you and make your intentions heard.

❈ Don't be afraid to make a change if you are unhappy in your current job.

❈ Visualize your ideal career often in order to increase your chances of attracting what you want.

Physical Activity

Moving your body gives you energy, promotes digestion and circulation, and helps you maintain a healthy weight. When it comes to maintaining a healthy lifestyle moving your body is a must, as it rejuvenates your mind, body, and spirit.

Key Points for Moving Your Body

❈ Working out boosts your energy and stamina. The more tired you feel, the more you need to move your body.

❈ Start with small steps, so you gradually build up your new habit and endurance.

❁ Build up a new exercise routine based on an already existing habit, if you want the new habit to stick.

❁ Try to move your body at least 20 minutes a day, even if all you do is walk or climb the stairs.

❁ Move your body naturally, by opting for walking instead of driving when possible. You don't need to wear sneakers to move your body.

❁ Working out is not a chore, but a lifestyle. Try to adopt it yourself, too, and enjoy the benefits of living a healthy-zesty lifestyle!

Purpose

This is the last step in the program that really brings everything full circle.

Your purpose is what helps you go through life with ease and the reason why you keep going.

Without a purpose, you have no idea where you are going. You have no target and no way of knowing if you succeeded. Just like navigating without a map and final destination. You will never know you arrived, as you never knew where you were heading to begin with.

So, now, at the end of our journey together I invite you to reflect over your why again. What do you really want? Why do you want to have more energy and feel healthy and zesty? What's on the horizon for you?

Remember that feeling healthy and vibrant is just the enabler, not the destination. So, where are you heading?

You are now closer to having the energy and clarity to define your purpose, the life of your dreams. There is nothing stopping you now! It's your chance to go after what you truly and deeply want. Go for what you always wanted but you couldn't go after because you were pulled back by fatigue, lack of motivation, hope, and purpose. You now know that you have the strength within you to chase your dreams and you owe this to yourself.

CONCLUSION

Bringing It All Into Balance

Just remember that you are enough already, you just need to get in touch with your real self, your deepest desires and commit to nourishing yourself not only with clean, whole foods but with clean thoughts, self-love, healthy relationships, satisfying work, gentle exercise and clear purpose. Once you understand the importance of all these factors for living a healthy and vibrant life and take steps toward bringing them all into balance, your life will change for the better. Maybe for the first time in a long time, you will start feeling awake and present like a veil has come off your eyes and you can actually see. See the beauty of your life, even if challenges come your way at times. You will now be more prepared to face them and turn them into opportunities.

As a result of the changes made, you will experience clear thinking, energy, and excitement, which is what will help you move forward with purpose and reach your ultimate goals, whatever those are. It is your chance for living the life you were meant to live and becoming the best version of yourself! Your Healthy-Zesty Life! Isn't that what we all want?

We only have one life to live, so we better make the best of it!

Visit www.healthyzesty.com for even more information!

Go to www.healthyzesty.com/3-day-healthy-zesty-jumpstart-menu to download your 3-day menu!

This book was inspired by my own healing journey coupled with my learning experience at the Institute for Integrative Nutrition® (IIN®) where I received my training in holistic wellness and health coaching. IIN® offers a truly comprehensive Health Coach Training Program that invites students to deeply explore the things that are most nourishing to them. From the physical aspects of nutrition and eating wholesome foods that work best for each individual person, to the concept of *Primary Food*[31] – the idea that everything in life including our spirituality, career, relationships, and fitness contribute to our inner and outer health - IIN® helped me deepen my holistic health and wellness knowledge and reach optimal health and balance. This inner journey unleashed the passion that compelled me to share my experience, my aha moments and inspire others for living a healthy and vibrant life. I invite you to learn more about the Institute for Integrative Nutrition® and explore how the Health Coach Training Program can help you transform your life. Feel free to contact me to hear more about my personal experience at [www.healthyzesty.com].

---

31 © 2005 Integrative Nutrition Inc. (used with permission)

For more support beyond the book, check out my website:

www.healthyzesty.com

And don't miss a single thing! Sign up for my weekly newsletter to receive healthy-zesty tips and recipes directly to your inbox. It's all on my website!

Did you enjoy my book? I would love your honest review!

Interested in having Camelia speak at your next event?

Camelia's passion for helping others improve their health and vitality through healthy eating and balanced living goes way beyond this book. Aside from providing private and group health coaching she is also on a mission to spread the word about the importance of a healthy gut for overall well-being by serving as a keynote speaker for various events.

For more information or to hire Camelia for your next keynote or event, email cameliapanati@healthyzesty.com

Testimonials

I don't have enough words to recommend Camelia's book to any woman! Even to those who don't think they have any problem. It's very easy to become addicted to work when you have a deep passion for your work. It's easy to replace a few hours of sleep with a few hours of more pleasant work. But eventually the enthusiasm will turn into exhaustion. Camelia's book taught me how to take care of myself, be healthier and more productive in my work. I feel that I am really lucky that I could benefit from her knowledge.

~ Geta Grama

Founder of Geta's Quilting Studio

What I love about "Your Healthy Zesty Life" is that it not only paints the picture on how to change specific things in my life to make me feel better, but it also provides the details and support to get started. This is exactly what I needed to take the first step to a healthier lifestyle and abundant energy. Passion, inner peace and love are what inspires this book!

~ Billi Jo Wright

SVP Partnership Development & Client Management

There is no better knowledge than first-hand knowledge and that's exactly what you get from Camelia Panati. Her experiene is one that we can all benefit from.

~Hailey Dolan, Designer

NO GUTS, NO GLORY...! A fascinating insight into how Camelia revitalized her life through a healthy lifestyle metamorphosis. This is excellent reading for anyone suffering chronic fatigue and searching for alternative solutions. The principles of good health outlined in this book are certain to bring vibrant energy and inner serenity back into the lives of many readers.

~ Terence Moraczewski, MD

Camelia Panati's book hits the spot for anyone starving to regain the energy or thirsting for the knowledge to discover wellness. Highly recommended reading for any patient that presents for perpetual tiredness with no obvious medical explanation.

~ David Hall, MD

What delicious food for thought 'Chef' Camelia has served us with her effervescent writing! This novel is a must for all women over-worked by obligations but undernourished by the rules to a happier, healthier, holistic life!

~ Laila Salts, MD

This magnificent book is not only a useful tool to identify the need for change, but also a mirror for the whole course of your life. It makes you understand how you created everything that you are and it pulls you by the hand to get you out of all comfort zones. If you dare to read it, it ends up reading you!

~ Melya Andra, Soprano

Food Journal

Day I (Date:)

Breakfast
_____
_____
_____
_____

Lunch
_____
_____
_____
_____
_____

Snack
_____
_____
_____
_____

Dinner
_____
_____
_____
_____
_____

How Much Water Did I Drink?
Circle How Many 8 oz. Glasses

1   2   3   4   5   6   7   8

How I Feel Today				
Mood	Digestion	Energy	Headache	Other
Breakfast				
Lunch				
Snack				
Dinner				

How Did I Feel Overall?
Circle One Option Below

EXCELLENT   GREAT   OK   NOT TOO GOOD   BAD

Day 2 (Date:)

Breakfast

Lunch

Snack

Dinner

How Much Water Did I Drink?
Circle How Many 8 oz. Glasses

1   2   3   4   5   6   7   8

How I Feel Today				
Mood	Digestion	Energy	Headache	Other
Breakfast				
Lunch				
Snack				
Dinner				

How Did I Feel Overall?
Circle One Option Below

EXCELLENT   GREAT   OK   NOT TOO GOOD   BAD

Day 3 (Date:)

Breakfast

_____
_____
_____
_____
_____

Lunch

_____
_____
_____
_____
_____

Snack

_____
_____
_____
_____
_____

Dinner

_____
_____
_____
_____
_____

How Much Water Did I Drink?
Circle How Many 8 oz. Glasses

1   2   3   4   5   6   7   8

How I Feel Today				
Mood	Digestion	Energy	Headache	Other
Breakfast				
Lunch				
Snack				
Dinner				

How Did I Feel Overall?
Circle One Option Below

EXCELLENT   GREAT   OK   NOT TOO GOOD   BAD

Day 4 (Date:)

Breakfast

Lunch

Snack

Dinner

How Much Water Did I Drink?
Circle How Many 8 oz. Glasses

1   2   3   4   5   6   7   8

How I Feel Today				
Mood	Digestion	Energy	Headache	Other
Breakfast				
Lunch				
Snack				
Dinner				

How Did I Feel Overall?
Circle One Option Below

EXCELLENT   GREAT   OK   NOT TOO GOOD   BAD

Day 5 (Date:)

Breakfast

_____
_____
_____
_____
_____

Lunch

_____
_____
_____
_____
_____

Snack

_____
_____
_____
_____

Dinner

_____
_____
_____
_____
_____

How Much Water Did I Drink?
Circle How Many 8 oz. Glasses

1   2   3   4   5   6   7   8

How I Feel Today				
Mood	Digestion	Energy	Headache	Other
Breakfast				
Lunch				
Snack				
Dinner				

How Did I Feel Overall?
Circle One Option Below

EXCELLENT   GREAT   OK   NOT TOO GOOD   BAD

Day 6 (Date:)

Breakfast

Lunch

Snack

Dinner

How Much Water Did I Drink?
Circle How Many 8 oz. Glasses

1   2   3   4   5   6   7   8

How I Feel Today				
Mood	Digestion	Energy	Headache	Other
Breakfast				
Lunch				
Snack				
Dinner				

How Did I Feel Overall?
Circle One Option Below

EXCELLENT   GREAT   OK   NOT TOO GOOD   BAD

Day 7 (Date:)

Breakfast

Lunch

Snack

Dinner

How Much Water Did I Drink?
Circle How Many 8 oz. Glasses

1   2   3   4   5   6   7   8

How I Feel Today				
Mood	Digestion	Energy	Headache	Other
Breakfast				
Lunch				
Snack				
Dinner				

How Did I Feel Overall?
Circle One Option Below

EXCELLENT   GREAT   OK   NOT TOO GOOD   BAD

References

Bassil, K L, et al. www.cfp.ca. October 2007. September 2016.

Chopra Center. www.chopra.com. 2016. September 2016.

Dinicolantonio, James J. and Sean C. Lucan. www.nytimes.com. 22 December 2014. September 2016.

DrWeil.com. www.drweil.com. 15 September 2016. September 2016.

FoxNews.com. foxnews.com/health/. 24 November 2013. 15 September 2016.

Hadhazy, Adam. http://www.scientificamerican.com/article/gut-second-brain/. 12 February 2010. September 2016.

Keefe, Bernadette. http://blog.centerforinnovation.mayo.edu. 7 April 2016. September 2016.

Lipman, Frank. www.drfranklipman.com. 10 February 2014. September 2016.

Murray, Michael. "The Condensed Encyclopedia of Healing Foods." Murray, Michael, Joseph Pizzorno and Lara Pizzorno. n.d.

National Geographic. "Discovering the Blue Zones Solution." National Geographic. Blue Zones. The Science of Living Longer (2016): 9.

Rosenthal, Joshua. Integrative Nutrition. Feed Your Hunger for Health and Happiness). Joshua Rosenthal, 2014.

Taylor, Nicole Fallon. www.businessnewsdaily.com. 15 January 2016.

September 2016.

www.ingramcontent.com/pod-product-compliance
Lightning Source LLC
Chambersburg PA
CBHW071357310526
45789CB00020B/408